THE HEALTHY DEVIANT

THE HEALTHY DEVIANT

A Rule Breaker's Guide to Being
Healthy in an Unhealthy World

Pilar Gerasimo

 North Atlantic Books

Published by
North Atlantic Books
Berkeley, California

Cover art and interior illustrations by Pilar Gerasimo (www.pilargerasimo.com)
Book design by Brian Johnson, Box 86, LLC (www.box8ighty6ix.com)
Healthy Deviant logotype: Andrei Lodiyr (www.lodiyr.ru)
Just Another Hand Font: Astigmatic One Eye Typographic Institute

Printed in Canada

The Healthy Deviant: A Rule Breaker's Guide to Being Healthy in an Unhealthy World is sponsored and published by the Society for the Study of Native Arts and Sciences (dba North Atlantic Books), an educational nonprofit based in Berkeley, California, that collaborates with partners to develop cross-cultural perspectives, nurture holistic views of art, science, the humanities, and healing, and seed personal and global transformation by publishing work on the relationship of body, spirit, and nature.

North Atlantic Books' publications are available through most bookstores. For further information, visit our website at www.northatlanticbooks.com or call 800-733-3000.

MEDICAL DISCLAIMER: The following information is intended for general information purposes only. Individuals should always see their health care provider before administering any suggestions made in this book. Any application of the material set forth in the following pages is at the reader's discretion and is his or her sole responsibility.

Library of Congress Cataloging-in-Publication Data

Names: Gerasimo, Pilar, 1967- author.
Title: The healthy deviant : a rule breaker's guide to being healthy in an
    unhealthy world / Pilar Gerasimo.
Description: Berkeley : North Atlantic Books, 2020. | Includes
    bibliographical references.
Identifiers: LCCN 2019032767 (print) | LCCN 2019032768 (ebook) | ISBN
    9781623174255 (trade paperback) | ISBN 9781623174262 (ebook)
Subjects: LCSH: Deviant behavior. | Self-care, Health.
Classification: LCC HM811 .G43 2020 (print) | LCC HM811 (ebook) | DDC
    302.5/42--dc23
LC record available at https://lccn.loc.gov/2019032767
LC ebook record available at https://lccn.loc.gov/2019032768

1 2 3 4 5 6 7 8 9 MARQUIS 25 24 23 22 21 20

This book includes recycled material and material from well-managed forests. North Atlantic Books is committed to the protection of our environment. We print on recycled paper whenever possible and partner with printers who strive to use environmentally responsible practices.

For Dad, who taught us to ask:
Why do we live the way we do?

And for Mom, who taught us to ask:
How could we live more the way we'd like to?

Wink, Wink, Nudge, Nudge

On many occasions over the past few years, when I'd tell people I was writing a book about "healthy deviance," they'd look at me with raised eyebrows. Then they'd kind of chuckle or grin at me in that way that says, "*Ha ha*, so it sounds like *you're* up to something fun, eh? Wink, wink, nudge, nudge."[1]

I didn't have the heart to tell most of those people that I was writing this book for one important (and not wonderfully fun or racy) reason: *Currently, we live in a culture that produces more unhealthy, unhappy people than healthy, happy ones.*

In fact, right now, the unhealthy-to-healthy ratio is arguably running about a hundred to one. I'll lay out my rationale for that statistic in chapter 1, but here's one thing I can tell you for sure: If you are currently a healthy and happy person in today's United States of America (or in any one of a growing number of countries now following our lead), you represent a tiny and shrinking minority. *You are, statistically speaking, an endangered species.*

I know, that is way less sexy than all the winkers and nudgers might have hoped. And if you bought this book thinking it was about, um, something else, I'm sorry to disappoint you. In my mind, though, these facts do raise a rather captivating question: *What kind of society makes being healthy and happy so difficult that only a tiny, single-digit percentage of its population can hope to pull it off?*

The answer is self-evident: A sick society. And within a sick society—one where chronic illness, obesity, drug dependence, anxiety, and depression are rapidly becoming the prevailing norms—what does it mean to be one of the few who bucks those unhealthy odds? It means that you have to be prepared to successfully resist your society's standard way of doing business. You have to oppose its rules and defy its conventions. You have to make all kinds of inconvenient and unpopular choices. You have to become a sort of renegade freak—or at least be willing to think and act like one some of the time.

The great news is that this does not require superhuman willpower, single-digit body-fat percentages, buns of steel, or an endless parade of boneless, skinless chicken breasts. What it does require: a willingness to toss some official-looking rule books out the window, to suspend some self-torpedoing beliefs and assumptions, and to begin doing some things ... differently.

That starts with understanding one basic, disturbing fact: *If you aren't breaking the rules, you're probably breaking yourself.*

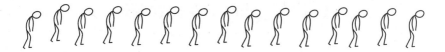

Over the past fifty years or so, breaking ourselves is exactly what most of us have been doing. We've either been following our culture's paths of least resistance (processed foods, sedentary screen time, reliance on symptom-suppressing drugs), or we've been getting dragged along by its punishing health-improvement prescriptions (unachievable perfect-body ideals, fussy diets, overwhelming exercise routines). Or, worse, we've been staggering around, exhausted and inflamed, doing all of the above.

In the process, we have been inadvertently playing into the hands of the very systems that are breaking us down. Clearly, we have to stop doing that—but rescinding our complicity with the unhealthy dominant culture is easier said than done. Moving away from our society's preprogrammed defaults requires busting out of well-worn ruts, swimming against powerful tides. All of which requires energy, attention, and resilience that most busy, exhausted, chronically overwhelmed people simply do not have to spare.

All forms of social deviance—even the healthy, positive kind—carry unspoken costs and risks. And that's one big, wildly underappreciated reason why, despite their best efforts, the vast majority of people who chase health and happiness in our culture don't ever attain them. Yet somehow, against all odds, a few healthy oddballs manage to pull it off. Some of them even make it look easy. The question is: *How?*

This book represents my best attempt to answer that question. Drawing on what I've learned over the course of two decades as a health journalist, as well as my own experience as a lifelong health seeker, I share the unlikely means by which a small but growing number of bright-spot outliers are managing to pull off the seemingly impossible—and how you can, too.

The way of the Healthy Deviant starts with taking a step back, dusting yourself off, and seeing through fresh eyes the true nature of the health-seeking quest in front of you. That means letting go of pointless self-recrimination, recognizing that your genes and current environment are an evolutionary mismatch of almost unfathomable proportions, and that your bodily systems were simply never wired to work the way you are asking them to work today.

Next, you'll learn to rise to that challenge and to navigate that quest more skillfully, growing stronger, clearer, and more confident as you go. This involves reclaiming and reframing your own Healthy Deviant story, and (if you choose) embarking on your own 14-Day Healthy Deviant Adventure.

During the course of that adventure, you'll develop some essential Nonconformist Competencies, practice some delightful Renegade Rituals, and build some game-changing Healthy Deviant Survival Skills. The final step is forging your own Healthy Deviant identity—one that's largely impervious to dominant-culture ills and illusions.

Embracing Healthy Deviance at this level requires acknowledging your present circumstances while simultaneously redefining yourself as a sovereign individual. It means choosing to be animated rather than oppressed by the predominantly unhealthy default choices that surround you.

That's the Healthy Deviant Way. And while not an instant fix, it actually works a whole lot faster and more reliably than most health-improvement strategies that promise instant results. It's also a whole lot more fun.

Is There Science Behind This?

I'm so glad you asked. Yes. Plenty. While I have not littered the text with endless notes, I have tried to serve up enough of a science-based bread-crumb trail that anyone interested in going deeper can do so. When applicable, I've referenced the researchers and scientists whose work has most informed my own. In some cases, I've referenced specific studies, books, articles, or websites. In others, I've simply noted larger bodies of knowledge and schools of thought, figuring you can google your way to more data, if you wish.

When all of that science and research is synthesized, though, the Healthy Deviant approach rests on one very basic, solid, science-supported thesis: *Faced with a serious, high-stress challenge, an aware, energized, and resilient person stands a much better chance of coping than a distracted, depleted, and fragile one.*

Research experiments have repeatedly demonstrated that under conditions requiring us to exert a great deal of self-control or endure a significant level of stress, humans experience a rapid depletion of attention, cognitive capacity, and what we think of as "willpower." Translation: No matter how healthy your intentions, confronted with a long-enough stream of pressures, frustrations, and temptations, eventually you will cave and take the path of least resistance.

This is a phenomenon (sometimes called "ego depletion," a topic I'll address in chapter 2) that virtually all of us have experienced firsthand. And no wonder: For most of us, "conditions that require us to exert a great deal of self-control or endure a significant level of stress" pretty much describes the bulk of *our everyday lives.*

Because escape from that set of circumstances has seemed largely impossible, most people have become habituated to some form of chronic, low-grade misery. They willingly endure ongoing discomfort, coping as best they can. This sets them up for another psychological phenomenon known as "learned helplessness" (which I'll cover in chapter 3). Clearly, this is not a state that predisposes one toward conscious, empowered choice.

Okay, so that's the bad news. But here's the good news: Research shows that recognizing you're the subject of an experiment tends to alter that experiment's outcomes—typically in your favor. Once you're aware of the experiment's conditions and your role within it, you become more cognizant both of your own initial instincts and behaviors and of the full range of options available to you. That means that instead of going along with the research agenda, you're inclined to make choices that serve your own best interests. In other words, rather than being an unwitting participant in the experiment, you become an active shaper (or, more to the point, *disruptor*) of it.

This is why researchers generally endeavor not to let subjects know the parameters and purpose of the experiments they are running. They know that it would totally skew the results. Avoiding that sort of interference is all well and good in the lab, but when it comes to the life-and-death circumstances we're all facing now, I think we can agree this experiment could use some skewing in our favor.

Right, so here's the deal:

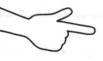

Before you embark on any health-motivated diet, exercise, or self-help program, it helps to understand the nature of the real-world context in which that effort is taking place.

It helps to instill the practices and perspectives that give you the best possible advantage in dealing with our crazy-culture dynamics. It helps to acquire the skills that empower you to operate successfully within them.

That, in essence, is the strategy behind the Healthy Deviant approach. Many of its tactics amount to jujitsu moves—the use of artful, subtle, low-effort shifts that achieve major leverage and some surprisingly big results. Its larger promise lies in making the whole process of getting healthier more fun, easeful, and rewarding than whatever you've been doing (or dreading doing) for ages.

So, just for now, let's set aside all the struggle and self-denial. Let's ease up on the self-blame and the "shoulds" and the impossible ideals. Instead, let's take a closer look at what is really going on in this weird, constraining experiment we find ourselves living daily. And let's reframe the act of being healthy in an unhealthy world as a creative, heroic, and profoundly exciting act of social rebellion. Because, as all Healthy Deviants know (wink, wink, nudge, nudge), that's precisely what it is.

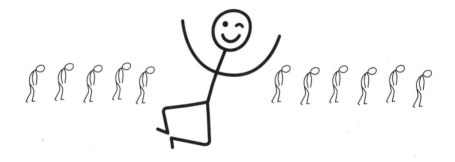

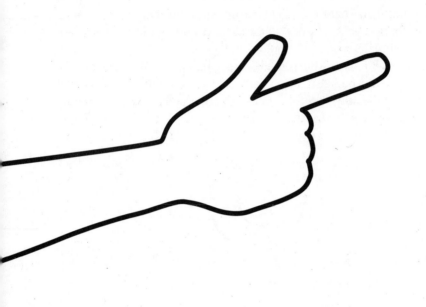

Healthy Deviants Wanted

FOR DARING ADVENTURE

Currently seeking bold, adventuresome,

health-motivated individuals

to buck deadly trends and

disrupt unhealthy social norms.

Must be willing to defy convention,

question authority and absurdity,

sidestep conformity,

and master a wide variety of

healthy-person skills, including

the art of illuminating the best within them.

No experience necessary.

Training provided.

Desire to explore and

willingness to experiment helpful.

Generous benefits package includes

increased energy and resilience,

radiant health and vitality,

and a dramatically expanded sense

of what's possible.

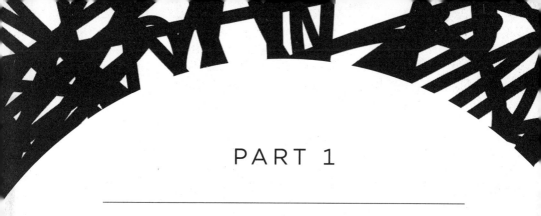

PART 1

The Crazy That Passes for Normal

It is no measure of health to be
well adjusted to a profoundly sick society.
—JIDDU KRISHNAMURTI

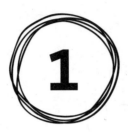

Welcome, Rule Breaker

Without deviation, progress is not possible.
—FRANK ZAPPA

Hi. Thanks for showing up. I was hoping you would. I've been wanting to talk to you about something important. Something urgent, actually.

First, though, how are you? No, really, I want to know: *How are you*? I'm concerned about you. I recognize that look. A bit frazzled, a bit tired, maybe a bit frantic, but wearing a tight little smile that says "Nothing to see here! Everything's just fine!"

Hmm. I wonder. Is everything fine with you? Truly?

I ask because, frankly, a lot of the people I know aren't doing all that great right now. I'm not sure if you've heard, but a lot of our friends have been getting really sick. Some are dying.

Hey, I realize you are probably busy, stressed out, and dealing with a thousand different things, and the last thing I want to do is add to your list of burdens. But I thought you'd want to know. Or maybe I just really felt like I needed to tell you. You're in a rush? Okay, maybe it's better if I show you …

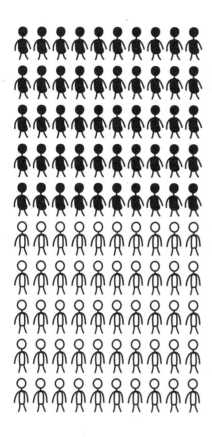

50%

of U.S. adults are diagnosed with chronic illnesses.

Source: Centers for Disease Control
https://www.cdc.gov/chronicdisease/overview

I know. *What?!*

But yes. According to the Centers for Disease Control, more than half of us have been diagnosed with a chronic disease. Many of us have more than one. And it's likely a great many more of us are chronically ill and just haven't been diagnosed yet.

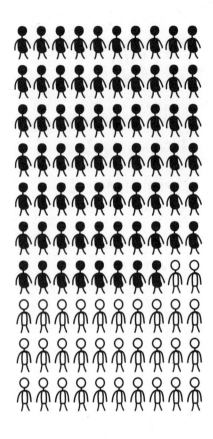

68%
are overweight or obese.

Source: Centers for Disease Control
https://www.cdc.gov/nchs/fastats/obesity-overweight.htm

One important contributing factor to all that chronic illness is metabolic disruption. Right now, two-thirds of us are carrying around excess weight. This increases our risk of many chronic diseases, especially inflammatory, metabolic, and hormonal conditions like type 2 diabetes, heart disease, autoimmune disorders, Alzheimer's, and many types of cancer.

Being significantly overweight can also make us far more likely to feel fatigued and depressed, to sleep poorly, and to suffer from arthritis and infertility, among many other life-limiting conditions. And all of those things can significantly increase the likelihood of our being prescribed pharmaceutical drugs, as more than two-thirds of us are today.

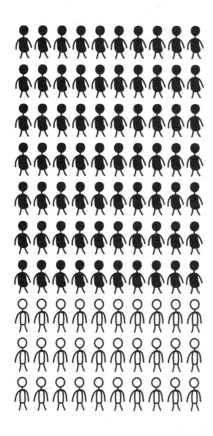

70%
are taking at least one prescription drug.

Source: Mayo Clinic Proceedings
http://www.mayoclinicproceedings.org/article/S0025-6196(13)00357-1/abstract

Two thirds? Again, yes. I realize it sounds crazy, but a 2013 study published in the *Mayo Clinic Proceedings* suggests that about 70 percent of adults in the United States have been prescribed a pharmaceutical drug in the past year. A 2017 Consumer Reports study suggests that about 55 percent are taking at least one prescription drug daily. And keep in mind, many people are taking multiple drugs each day. For folks over sixty, the average number is *five*.

The most commonly prescribed daily drugs are for high blood pressure, cholesterol, depression, digestive problems, and other conditions predominantly driven by lifestyle-related factors. All prescription drugs have side effects and can interact in ways that negatively affect both the body and the mind.

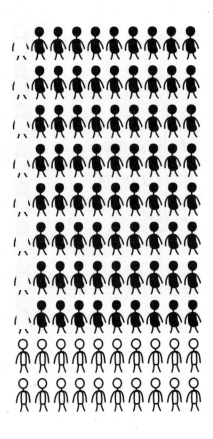

80%
are mentally or emotionally "not flourishing."

Source: National Institutes of Health
https://www.ncbi.nlm.nih.gov/pmc/articles/PMC3477942

Maybe all that prescription drug use has something to do with the fact that, according to research published in the *Journal of Health and Social Behavior,* about 80 percent of us aren't thriving mentally or emotionally.[2] Instead, the vast majority of adults in the United States are struggling with some level of anxiety or depression, suffering from chronic or post-traumatic stress, dealing with attention or mood disorders, or just feeling kind of blah. In the words of psychology researcher Barbara Fredrickson, PhD, they are "just getting by" or, worse, "leading lives of quiet despair."[3]

Like I said, it seems like most people we know aren't doing all that great. And, unfortunately, based on our current health habits, it doesn't look like things are going to be getting better anytime soon.

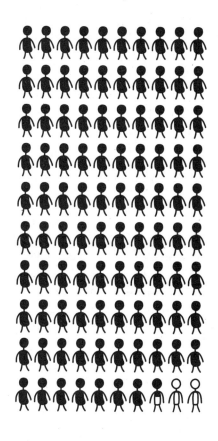

97.3%

not maintaining
healthy habits:
- decent nutrition
- adequate exercise
- not smoking
- healthy body
  composition

Source: Mayo Clinic Proceedings
http://www.ncbi.nlm.nih.gov/pubmed/26906650

Yep. Research published in the *Mayo Clinic Proceedings* reveals that 97.3 percent of us aren't managing to maintain even four of the most basic habits required for long-term health.[4] The four habits considered in this research were:

- Eating a reasonably balanced, nutritious diet (based on a week's worth of notoriously unreliable self-reported data and measured against the USDA's hotly debated Healthy Eating Index).

- Getting "adequate" activity (a weekly total of 150 minutes of moderate to vigorous exercise, as tracked by an accelerometer).

- Maintaining a healthy body composition (under 20 percent body fat for men; under 30 percent for women, as measured by a DEXA scan).

- Not smoking (confirmed by a blood test).

It's wild to think that only a single-digit percentage of U.S. adults (2.7 percent!) is managing to do these essential, self-preserving things. But wait, it gets *worse,* because the research looking at those four supposedly basic health habits did not even begin to consider a number of *other* lifestyle factors that studies have shown to be equally important (or potentially even more important) to our health. Those factors include:

- Getting enough high-quality sleep.

- Effectively managing or moderating stress.

- Maintaining strong, supportive social connections.

The science is clear: Regardless of how well you eat, and even if you exercise regularly, don't smoke, and maintain a healthy body composition, if you don't get enough deep sleep, don't manage stress, and don't have a supportive community, you are going to be at much higher risk for getting sick and depressed. You are also dramatically more likely to die early.

Okay, so if we were to add those three additional factors to the original list of four key health habits, how many people do you think would be reliably doing *all seven of them*? How many could we reasonably categorize as healthy, happy, and (by virtue of their self-preserving lifestyle habits) on track to stay that way for the foreseeable future?

It's impossible to say for sure, because that research hasn't been done yet. And frankly, it probably never will be, because there are just too many complex factors for a single, well-designed, statistically significant study to accurately assess. But if I had to hazard an educated guess, I'd say it is probably less than 1 percent of the U.S. adult population. That would look something like this:

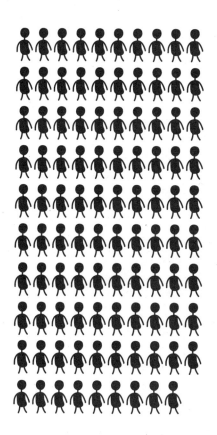

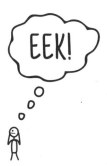

Maybe 1% healthy, happy, and on track to stay that way?

EEK!

Data or no data, what we know for certain is that way too few of us have a decent shot at maintaining a high level of health, happiness, and vitality in this culture. And if research on the current health state of our children is any indication, the next generation is not projected to fare much better.

But let's get back to you and your right-now reality. *How are you doing?* Really, truly—without all the look-good, sound-good filters. How's your energy these days? What's going on with your skin? Your gut?

I know it's awkward and a little uncomfortable for me to be probing like this. I've already asked you that question—*how are you?*—three times, whereas social custom clearly dictates that I should ask it only once. Social custom also says I definitely shouldn't be getting so personal. We both know how this works:

- I ask the rhetorical question, "How are you?" (not really expecting an honest answer).

- Then you reply with the rhetorical answer, "Fine" (regardless of how you are actually doing). ·

- And then we go our separate ways. Easy. Done.

That's what's known as a *social norm*. I'm breaking one right now to make a point. But my annoying, awkward, socially inappropriate question also has a legitimate objective, and that's to get us to a truth we might both otherwise be inclined to avoid out of politeness and propriety.

Clearly, social norms serve a purpose. They simplify our lives in a thousand ways. They dictate proper action, and help us know what to expect. They bind us together and beat back chaos. But they can also unnecessarily constrain and disserve us. They can lead us astray. They can put us to sleep. They can make us deny what's true about ourselves and the world around us. They can make us forget who we are and why we are here.

Well, to hell with that. This is a book about waking up and showing up and remembering what we're really made of. It's a book about taking back the sense of vitality and freedom that is our birthright. This is a book about breaking the rules that are breaking us. So, I'm going to ask you again: *How are you?* And I'm going to keep on asking. You can run away or go back to sleep if you want, but I'd rather you didn't. I'd rather you stayed here with me. I'd rather we told each other the truth.

Here's a truth I've learned the hard way: Just as this brand of intimate conversation between strangers breaks with some well-established social norms, so do a great many of the other things you might choose to do in the name of your own health and well-being. That includes what you do or do not choose to eat, as well as how and when you choose to move, sleep, work, rest, and play. It could also include how you manage your energy, attention, mood, money, time, relationships, health care, media, and view of the world.

Do enough of those things differently from most of the people around you, and at some point, you are going to get weird looks. You are going to get pushback. I'm guessing that you probably already are. And here's why: In the context of a predominantly unhealthy culture, making healthy choices requires deviating from widely accepted expectations. It requires steering around a slew of well-established social norms. In other words, it requires deviance. So, in essence:

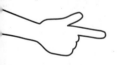 Being healthy = being socially deviant.

Regularly engaging in any kind of social deviance is a challenging proposition. Breaking from society's prevailing norms and conventions (even when your life depends on it) is rarely easy. In fact, it often feels like an awkward, inconvenient, downright demoralizing slog. On the other hand, it can also be a liberating, exhilarating, wildly rewarding adventure—*if* you grasp what you're up against, and you know what you're doing. Which, with this book in hand, you will.

Deviance, Reconsidered

There's a reason I get so many "wink, wink, nudge, nudge" responses when I mention Healthy Deviance: The term *deviant* sounds naughty. That's because, historically, it has been applied to all sorts of troublemakers and outcasts. It's a term we've typically reserved for criminals, addicts, lunatics, and people with peculiar predilections. It's a term we like to slap on people we disapprove of, people who stubbornly refuse to conform—a category that has, over the course of history, included everybody from artists and homosexuals to spiritual leaders and civil-rights heroes.

In reality, a deviant is simply someone who doesn't go along with society's status-quo norms and standards. Most of us adhere to our culture's social norms most of the time (that's what makes them social norms). We do this because, in many cases, those norms make good sense. As noted, conforming to societal expectations makes it easier to get along with others and to get things done without a lot of hassle.

Generally, we don't do a deep analysis of the social norms we've grown up with. We simply comply with them, because a lifetime of conditioning has predisposed us to doing so automatically. By the time we are adults, most of us no longer give our culture's norms a second thought.

A great many social norms, like waving back when somebody waves at you, are just good manners. Saying "fine" when somebody asks you how you are is pretty harmless, even if it's not entirely true. But what if some of your culture's most broadly accepted norms and social standards are undermining your health and making you miserable? What if you can plainly see that they are oppressing and killing off a bunch of people you love, messing with your community, your country, and maybe even putting your entire home planet at risk? Then, I would say, you might be wise to consider the way of the Healthy Deviant.

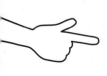

A Healthy Deviant is any person who willingly defies unhealthy norms and conventions in order to achieve a high level of vitality, resilience, and autonomy.

There is, interestingly, a branch of sociology dedicated to studying "positive deviance." This field of study investigates the bright-spot outliers who succeed in the midst of challenging situations. It attempts to discern how a scrappy few are managing to solve or work around intractable problems in ways that allow them to survive or thrive where most others do not. It explores how creative and resourceful individuals are figuring out solutions that experts, authorities, and large, official organizations have not. It studies and seeks to emulate those who are deviating, in good ways, from a not-so-good status quo.

Healthy Deviance is, in essence, a form of conscious, positive deviance. It's not a failure of social compliance. On the contrary, it's a badge of non-conformist courage.

If that notion appeals to you, let's be courageous together. Let's scrap the social rules for a moment and continue with the conversation we were having before. For real: *How are you doing in your body right now?* How is your heart feeling? How is your head faring? How is your spirit holding up? What is going on with you—not just on the surface, but as many layers deep as you can feel?

Now, listen.... Can you hear that? Can you feel that? A little twinge or buzz or wobble? A little shadow or pang or ache? Some dull heaviness? Fatigue? Or maybe just ... numb? Ah. Now we're getting somewhere. Now we are getting to the urgent part: *Your body is trying to tell you something.*

I want to help you to hear your body and dare to heed its genius. Even if you don't always like what it has to say. Even if our culture is encouraging you to ignore it, doubt it, and drown it out. I want you to know that you and your body are already doing a lot of things *right*. Whatever else might be going on for you at this time, whatever brand of frazzled, fatigued, inflamed, or less-than-awesome state you might be experiencing, the fact that you picked up this book (and are still reading it) tells me you are doing a whole lot better than most.

Look, maybe you are nothing like 97.3 percent of the population and never have been. Maybe you're already doing great. Maybe you've got the world on a healthy string, and everything is going your way. Maybe you really are an unbreakable badass. Maybe you have found a reliable way to give no f*cks and are cruising along with an enviable body composition and without a care in the world. Maybe you are impervious to our culture's many ills and are already helping others find their healthy way in our unhealthy world.

If that sounds like you, rock on. It is possible that I have nothing to offer you here except a Healthy Deviant high-five and a pat on the back. In which case, I say, *Way to go, friend. Travel safely, and Godspeed.*

But I wonder: When some thoughtful person pauses and asks you how you are doing—when they ask it like they really mean it, and then they wait, quietly, looking into your eyes with concern, searching your face for the truth—do you ever feel like, oh, I don't know, like maybe you're going to ... cry?

Or do you ever feel suddenly peevish and defensive, like you have to keep that well-meaning, concerned, and increasingly annoying person at a distance with a requisite "Fine!" just so you don't risk taking a breath and opening up and babbling on about all the things that you're worried about; all the things you're not getting to; the things that scare you, depress you, or enrage you; all the things you fear are not good enough, that will probably never be good enough, and that you feel helpless to fix; all the things that make you feel at the edge of your last frayed nerve?

I used to feel that way a lot of the time. Tight smiled. Hard eyed. Brittle. On the edge of tears or on the edge of blowing up or breaking down. Often, I couldn't even tell which. I just knew that I really dreaded being asked *how I was, really.* I so desperately needed to ask that question of myself and then get quiet and listen, but that was not something I was willing to do. I knew I wasn't going to like what I heard. Because the only honest answer I had at that time wasn't at all the *right* answer, which is to say, the *expected* answer, the *normal* answer, the *socially acceptable* answer: "Fine."

The truth was, I wasn't doing fine—not by a long stretch. Clearly, most of us are not doing fine right now. And even if you *are* currently doing "fine," I don't want you to settle for that. I don't want you to sign yourself over to that deadly brand of mediocrity. I want you to know that you don't have to. I want you to experience what it feels like to fully inhabit your body-mind and feel weirdly radiant, resilient, and good in your own skin. I want you to throw off the shackles of "fine" and "normal" and "okay" and leave them in the dust. I want you to abandon all the conventions and unquestioned choices that are causing you pain.

I'm not just talking about those obviously unhealthy mainstream choices, like eating fast food, drinking too much, and watching too much television.

I'm also talking about a lot of popular, culturally condoned health-improvement prescriptions, including a great many well-intended diet, exercise, and "healthy lifestyle" ideals. Because, while both unhealthy default choices and misguided health-improvement prescriptions can mess with your body-mind, the combination of the two is an unmitigated disaster—the kind capable of undermining the health of an entire population.

The way I see it, adhering to our society's default patterns and its unrealistic health-improvement prescriptions has gotten us trapped in a vitality-sucking downward spiral. Nobody official and authoritative is coming to save us. It's up to us to find our own way out. So here, conspiring together, that's what we're going to do. I'm going to share the unexpected, counterintuitive escape plan that worked for me, and I'm going to help you discover (i.e., hatch) a Healthy Deviant plan that works for you.

Inside the Body-Mind

The term body-mind is my preferred way of referring to the complex, interconnecting systems that link the brain and central nervous system to the rest of the body. Science has shown us, incontrovertibly, that within the human system, everything is connected: Brain and gut, gut and skin, emotion and biochemistry, biochemistry and microbiome, and from the microbiome back to the brain again. Body-mind is my inclusive, intersecting term for all of it. If you prefer to substitute some other term, feel free.

Just remember that the body and brain are not separate entities. The functions and cascading molecular byproducts of our thoughts and feelings (or anything that takes place in the domain of what we call our "heart and mind" or "spirit") cannot be strained out or handled separately from the rest of the physiological self.

Forewarned Is Forearmed

The most basic lesson of Healthy Deviance is one you likely already know from personal experience: Becoming and staying a healthy person in our unhealthy culture can feel ridiculously hard—at first, anyway. You can't just roll merrily along doing whatever's easy, fast, popular, and automatic. You can't follow the paths of least resistance. On the contrary, you have to maintain a certain level of vigilance and effort just to avoid getting sucked into the vortex of the dominant-culture machine. That's the machine that is currently messing with the health of 99 percent of adults in this country (and also a lot of our kids).

This leaves you with a stark choice:

Break the rules, or break yourself.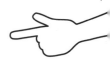

You'd think that would be an easy decision. Alas, it is not.

You probably already realize that you can't go along with the outrageous expectations this world throws at you and still stay sane. You probably know that you can't keep on chasing unrealistic body ideals, complying with all the conventional prescriptions, striving for all the socially condoned markers of success, and still stay healthy and happy.

But knowing this puts you in a tricky place. Because, while your inner rule breaker is the part most likely to pull you from the mire of the mixed-up world we are living in, it is also the part that will make you stand out from the crowd. It's that renegade aspect of your person that will surprise, confuse, alarm, disappoint, and anger others. It's the way-out-ahead part that will inspire judgment and jealousy. And that can feel dangerous—because often, frankly, it is.

Being out of the in-group always feels a little iffy, a little exposing, a little wrong. It carries a stigma—the kind that can cost you, hurt you, get you ditched or rolled or ridiculed by those whom you hold dear. We humans are herd animals. Somewhere deep down in our DNA, we know we need the company, support, and sustenance of others—not just to survive, but also to make our lives feel worth living.

Within every cell and fiber of our being, we carry an ancient memory, an evolutionary warning, a visceral, tribal truth, one that is constantly whispering, *You do not want to go this alone. You'd be crazy to even try.*

Well, I'm here to tell you that you are not alone, and you are not crazy. But feeling torn between two different types of self-preservation—one for physical survival and the other for social acceptance (which we intuitively understand is intrinsic to our physical survival)—can make you *feel* crazy. It can leave you feeling perennially anxious, confused, desperate, strung out, exhausted, and white-knuckle terrified, like you are rattling down the tarmac with your wheels about to come off. It can leave you feeling like no matter how hard you try, you just can't win. It can make you feel like you want to cry or explode or just plain give up.

The survivor in you is no fool. Given a clear opportunity to choose between dying a slow, miserable death or breaking some societal rules, you'll probably break some rules. At least I hope you will. That is a healthy instinct. Let's call it your Healthy Deviant instinct. The problem is, our culture actively discourages you from seeing that you *have* a choice. It dulls your healthy instincts, hides your healthy options, blocks your exits, and lulls you into complacency. It tricks and taunts and stupefies you. It convinces you that there's only one right way forward, and that is the way of the dominant-culture program.

How do I know all of this? Because that is the program I followed, right up until it broke me—literally. That breakage happened on an otherwise typical day, about two decades ago, in which I found myself hopelessly trapped between conflicting demands and ideals. Just another day in which I simply could not find a way to do everything I thought I had to do, be everything I thought I had to be, look how I thought I had to look, and achieve it all on a timeline and to standards that I deemed "good enough."

On some days like this I cried. On other days I ranted, fumed, or held my breath. And on this particular day, I stomped my foot. But I didn't just stomp it. *I stomped it in a fit of self-directed rage so powerful that I shattered one of my own bones.*

That's when my own Healthy Deviant instinct kicked in. That's when three Healthy Deviant truths slapped me in the face so hard that they woke me out of my mass-culture stupor and changed my life forever. For the better.

In part 2 of this book, I'll tell you the story of how all of that happened. I'm also going to ask you more about *your* story—the one that got you here, the one you're living now, and the one you still have left to write. First, though, I need to issue a few more words of warning.

- During the course of this book, I'm going to propose that you break a bunch of conventional rules, including some you might believe you should follow because they are "good for you."

- I'm also going to suggest you experiment with some unusual practices and points of view. You may have to let go of at least some of what you thought you knew and try some solutions that look too pleasant and easy to actually work (but they do).

- There is science behind these suggestions, but the only real way to know if some of these practices are effective for you will be to try them for yourself.

- This voyage will change you in ways that might surprise you—and others. To the extent you integrate this way of seeing and being, it will likely cause you to shift not just your perceptions but also your priorities, and eventually (I hope) many aspects of your life. You may find that all of this rubs some other people the wrong way.

If you can live with all of that, great. And if you aren't sure you can, that's okay, too. You don't have to do anything you don't want to do. I do, however, want you to know what you're in for. Because some of this could prove disruptive. At least I hope it will.

What's in Here, and What's Not

The goal of this book is to equip you to relate differently and more successfully to the unhealthy world around you, so that you have a better shot at pursuing whatever healthy goals matter to you.

This book will not try to magically mold you into a different size or shape. It won't insist you follow a particular diet, do a particular number of sets and reps, or burn a particular number of calories (more on all that in a minute). It presents no bikini-body makeovers, no six-pack-ab promises. It will not shame you into becoming someone you are not. Still, as noted, it might cause you to question some of your assumptions *(wait, no diet or exercise program?!),* as well as the habitual patterns and behaviors that others have come to expect from you.

Here's a quick look at this book's subversive yet commonsense premises, and what I'm hoping you'll take away from this body of work.

1. **Being a healthy, happy person in a predominantly unhealthy culture requires socially noncompliant (i.e., deviant) acts and attitudes.**

   If you live in a society that is wired up to produce mostly sick, stressed, semi-miserable people, it stands to reason that complying with that society's norms and conventions will eventually make you sick, stressed, and semi-miserable too. So, if you want to be healthy, you're going to have to start deviating from a bunch of unhealthy conventions. The problem is, all forms of social deviance are inherently un-automatic and counterintuitive. As a result, relatively few people are independently inclined to discover or embrace them. However, while the barriers to Healthy Deviance might initially seem daunting, they can be relatively easily overcome with the right strategies and know-how (which this book presents). And with even small-scale support from a merry band of fellow Healthy Deviants, over time, they become easier still.

2. **Our limited view of our present circumstances has caused us to misperceive the true nature of health problems, and to fall prey to a lot of ill-advised, counterproductive, and self-destructive coping strategies.**

We've long been encouraged to obsess about the symptoms of our personal health woes (excess weight, inflammatory disease, depression) rather than their root causes. We've also been programmed to accept our accumulating diagnoses as either a matter of genetic destiny, bad luck, or the result of our personal failings. Accordingly, we've been persuaded to accept a lot of short-sighted cures for our ever-expanding set of maladies—from ill-fated diets and workouts to pharmaceutical and surgical solutions—many of which wind up working directly *against* our sustainable health and happiness.

Meanwhile, what we have *not* been encouraged to see is that we are all, in effect, the subjects of a giant, uncontrolled experiment in evolutionary mismatch—the natural result of our environment and way of life changing much faster than our DNA can possibly adapt. This has made us vulnerable to a lot of pointless self-recrimination, leaving us discouraged, overwhelmed, and disempowered.

Once you see this booby-trapped terrain for what it is, it will be a whole lot easier to safely make your way out of it. You'll also understand why thriving in our historically unprecedented situation calls for something other than a simple shift of diet and exercise, or an upgrade of personal willpower.

3. **Repeated experiences of failure with ill-advised health-improvement tactics have led us to believe (wrongly) that our health issues are too difficult to overcome.**

From fussy, counterproductive, poorly conceived diets to exhausting, ineffective workouts, the struggle, deprivation, and lackluster results most people have experienced with conventional health-improvement prescriptions have led many to conclude that these health-seeking activities are simply not worth the effort they require. Others have decided that they are weak-willed and inherently flawed—simply not up to the task. In this way, conventional approaches to health and fitness often exacerbate and compound people's health struggles rather than relieving them.

The results have been widespread hopelessness, helplessness, exhaustion, self-loathing, and shame. Most people suffering from these feelings are understandably inclined to seek out pain-numbing, distraction, and "disease-management" strategies rather than navigating toward more satisfying, sustainable ways of living. Fortunately, it doesn't have to be that way.

4. **Healthy Deviance offers promising new means and methods for breaking free from these limiting conditions, and for helping others do the same.**

Societies are created by people, and people can change them. Some people (namely, Healthy Deviants) are particularly skilled at shifting them from the inside out. The Healthy Deviant framework (the essentials of which you'll learn in part 3 and get a chance to practice in part 4) gives you an exciting new way of seeing and relating to what previously seemed like insurmountable challenges. It gives you the exhilarating experience of perceiving clearly a bunch of previously obscured truths, and a means for moving beyond the grip of the oppressive, miserably limiting conditions too many of us have been suffering under for decades. It will help you find your chosen place in your own Healthy Deviant Hero's Journey, reunite you with your true, fierce self, and help you reclaim the vitality that is your birthright. It will also equip you with both the wisdom and moxie to help others—and when you are ready, you will likely feel compelled to do so.

And here we arrive at this book's central promise:

We can beat our sick society's unhealthy odds. But not by following its status-quo advice.

In some ways, this book is about an odd sort of disaster preparedness. It's not about planning for some big, dramatic, nightmarish event out there on the horizon; it's about figuring out how to more successfully navigate the real-life series of little disasters most of us face on a daily basis. That includes our society's prescribed approach to "diet and exercise."

The Problem with Diet and Exercise

As I was shopping this book around to agents and publishing houses, I got the same question again and again: *Is there a Healthy Deviant diet or a Healthy Deviant workout?* The answer was, and still is, a categorical no. Not because I'm not a big fan of healthy food and movement (I am). I'm just guessing that you've already tried a whole lot of diet and exercise programs and that most of them didn't work for you, or didn't work for very long.

And why didn't they work? Well, it could be those programs were of the poorly conceived, undernourishing, eat-less-and-exercise-more variety (which tend to fail everyone). Or it could be that those programs just weren't right for you, or not right for you at the time you tried them. Or it could be, just maybe, that you started out planning to follow each of those programs precisely, and then, well … didn't.

That happens to a lot of us. You know why? Because the world around us derails our healthy intentions with maddening consistency. The more most of us try to follow the conventional wisdom around diet and exercise, the *less* healthy and happy we get. The hungrier and more deprived we feel, the more inclined we are to say "to heck with this" and proceed to drown our sorrows in something awful.

Following conventional diet and exercise prescriptions coaxes most of us into doing a dance of one step forward and two steps back. And yet we live in a culture that strongly encourages us to just keep on dancing faster. It urges us to try *another* diet and *another* workout, while totally ignoring the fact that virtually none of what we are doing is working.

Consider this January 2018 article from the *Washington Post,* which reported that forty-five million Americans go on diets each year.[5] Note how it frames this fact: "It's unclear how successful those efforts are, though some experts say as few as 5 percent of dieters manage to keep the weight off long-term. Still, few would deny the impulse is a good one: About *70 percent of adults in the United States are overweight or obese."*

Um, wait. Let's just stop, rewind, and evaluate that for a moment. Could it possibly be, given those results (forty-five million going on diets annually with only a 5 percent success rate, and total of 70 percent of adults overweight or obese), that the impulse to go on yet another diet is *not* a good one?

This is the kind of crazy-making logic that our media spins out daily and that most of us accept unquestioningly, even though it makes little sense and is messing aggressively with our bodies and minds. And the popular dogma around exercise isn't much different. Here's another piece as reported by the *Washington Post,* this one from May 2017:[6]

> *Despite national guidelines that recommend 150 minutes of moderate activity each week for major health benefits plus strength work such as weights or push-ups, only about half of American adults get enough aerobic exercise, according to the Centers for Disease Control and Prevention.*
>
> *Nearly 30 percent get no physical activity in their spare time.*
>
> *Even when intentions are good, about half of people who start exercise programs drop out within the first six months, says Rodney Dishman, an exercise scientist at the University of Georgia in Athens. After two years, Dishman says, 80 percent have given up. Those numbers haven't budged over three decades of research, he adds.*

Again, all of this data would strongly suggest that what we are doing, and what we are being told to do by the powers that be, is clearly not working to our advantage. So here's my take: *While changes to our food and movement patterns certainly matter, they are not necessarily the best places to start.*

No matter how well intentioned our efforts in these domains, formal diet and exercise programs come packaged with all sorts of mental and emotional pressure (confusion, guilt, shame, anxiety, and self-denial). They require a lot of finagling, nit-picking, intensive self-regulation, and effort. Many come at a steep financial cost or prove otherwise inaccessible to a great many. Moreover, before we even begin, most of us are already so frazzled, depleted, and distracted, we simply aren't prepared to face the entrenched societal incentives and obstacles that have made those effort-intensive changes necessary in the first place.

As a result, diving headlong into such action-level prescriptions—even when they *are* scientifically sound—can quickly overwhelm even the most determined health seekers, further draining their energy and self-regulatory capacity and saddling them with an even longer string of perceived failures. So, for right now, I'm going to suggest that you go through the Healthy Deviant Adventure program at least once *without actively trying to change anything else that requires significant effort to change.*

Seriously, while you're reading this book, I'd like to invite you to not be "on a diet" or following a highly structured exercise program of any kind. Just eat what you choose to eat and move how you choose to move. Notice with interest what foods and forms of movement have found their way into your life, your space, your body. Notice the effect they have on your body-mind.

Of course, you could certainly decide to eat more whole foods and fewer processed ones (I'll offer some suggestions along those lines). You could decide to drink more water and fewer sweetened, caffeinated, or alcoholic beverages. You could decide to move your body more often and more delib- erately in ways that feel good to you. And if you do that, it will be interesting to notice the results. But for right now, it doesn't particularly matter. Because regardless of what you do, with enough attention on what you are *actually doing* (and why), I suspect you'll come to the same conclusion that I have:

To change your life for the healthier,
you don't just have to change your diet or your
workout; you have to shift your relationship
with the so-called normal world around you.

Yes, duh, of course, eating well and moving well are essential to your well-being. So is not smoking, getting enough sleep, managing stress, and forming supportive social connections. I'm guessing you know all of this al- ready. Because you've been probably told and lectured about it *ad nauseum*.

Here's what you may not have been told: If you are going to stand any realistic chance of being able to do *any* of those things, you must first prepare yourself to confront the forces of our unhealthy culture. You must learn to walk amidst them without being endlessly infected, subsumed, and jackrolled by them. Happily, this is precisely what embracing the way of the Healthy Deviant is going to help you do.

Still feeling game to give this Healthy Deviant thing a go? Good.

Let the rule breaking begin ...

How to Use This Book

Ha ha ha! Just kidding. Remember: *There are no rules!* You can use this book however you want (including as a gift to somebody else). This book is designed to meet you where you are and let you go at your own pace, according to your own appetites and instincts. Still, if you like being offered options, here are just few of the ways you might choose to proceed:

1. **Dive in:** Read the book from cover to cover, do all the exercises, and then complete the Healthy Deviant Adventure program as suggested. Use Daily Deviance Journal Pages, the Healthy Deviant Adventure Tracker, and any other tools and resources that seem helpful. See how that goes.

2. **Dabble:** Skim the book and let your instincts tell you what you most need to read first. Every day, pick one or more Renegade Rituals you feel like practicing, and combine them as you see fit. Every once in a while, open the book at random and see where your eyes land.

3. **Ramp up:** Read as much as you like for as long as you like. Do one Renegade Ritual daily for thirty days, two for the next thirty days, and three for the thirty days after that. Rotate in other activities as you feel ready.

4. **Let it sit:** I call this the "Talisman method," and it simply involves keeping the book near you as much as possible, ideally on some visible surface, where it can transmit its messages by osmosis. Let the title on the cover and spine speak to you from a distance and remind you of who you really are. The book might beckon to you on occasion. When you feel inclined, you can pick it up and hold it, and maybe proceed to the Dabble method from there.

Or invent your own method. However you do it is fine. Just know that if you keep reading, you may very well wind up seeing some things you can't easily unsee.

Seeing the Unseeable

This is your last chance. After this, there is no turning back.
You take the blue pill—the story ends, you wake up in your bed and
believe whatever you want to believe. You take the red pill—you
stay in Wonderland, and I show you how deep the rabbit hole goes.
Remember: All I'm offering is the truth. Nothing more.

—MORPHEUS (IN *THE MATRIX*)

In the classic 1999 film *The Matrix,* the mysterious Morpheus presents Neo, our naive and mystified protagonist, with two pills and a choice: Take the red pill and confront the reality of his situation (namely, that he is hooked up to a giant, illusion-producing machine that is sucking the life force out of him and most other humans), or take the blue pill and remain in deluded denial of that fact. It's an important decision, because, as Morpheus puts it, "There is no turning back."

In some ways, that is true of the perspectives I'll offer you here. Once you've seen this stuff, it's hard to unsee it. And yet, at the same time, it can be strangely hard to wrap your head around. Why? Because the central factor responsible for our most pressing health concerns is *so* big, *so* all-encompassing, and *so* in our faces that it has become largely invisible to us. That central factor is this:

Our most basic human needs are not being met during the course of what currently passes for "normal" daily life.

Even now, as I present this reality to you in large type, you may literally not be able or willing to "see" it. And even if you do see it, you may feel compelled to reject it or declare it obvious and therefore unimportant. You may elect to temporarily un-remember it—to barf up the red pill and swallow the blue pill instead.

Before you do, I invite you to read that statement again. Run it through your circuits. Argue with it, if you like. Here are a few questions that might come up for you, along with my quick answers:

Q: If our basic needs weren't being met, wouldn't we all be dead already?

A: We may not be dead yet, but we are certainly dying in droves for reasons we needn't be. Many of the top ten leading causes of death in the United States (heart disease, cancer, accidents, chronic lower respiratory disease, stroke, Alzheimer's disease, diabetes, influenza and pneumonia, kidney disease, and suicide) may be caused or directly influenced by lifestyle and environmental factors.[7] And rising rates of clinical depression, drug overdoses, suicide, and opioid addiction suggest that a lot of us may be feeling increasingly dead inside.

Q: What do you mean by "basic needs"?

A: By "basic needs," I mean our nonnegotiable requirements for surviving and thriving over the long term—things like nutritious food, clean water, freedom of movement, and safe shelter, as well as factors a few steps up on Maslow's hierarchy of needs, like belonging, connection, growth, and meaning. I'd also include access to natural sunlight and darkness; natural rhythms of waking and sleep; balanced cycles of exertion and rest; and time spent outdoors in natural environments. Because without these things, we begin a precipitous slide toward not-wellness. We also become more vulnerable to other things, including pathogens and infectious diseases of all kinds, as well as various forms of self-harm.

Q: **What do you mean by "what currently passes for 'normal' daily life"?**

A: I mean the typical Western-culture reality of living in a single-family home; working to make money and buy lots of things; commuting by mechanized means; spending most of our time indoors; regularly interacting with large institutions and bureaucratic systems; relying on automation and machines for most of what we want and need; consuming more than we create, being flooded by mass media and electric lights; being sedentary and chronically stressed; eating mostly processed and industrially prepared foods; and then using conventional diets, exercise programs, and medical interventions to deal with the fleet of intersecting problems (e.g., obesity, inflammation, chronic disease, depression, and anxiety) that predictably result from living that way.

Q: **Hey, wait, isn't this what the ancestral health and paleo or primal movements are all about?**

A: Yes—and no. Let's talk about that …

Getting Past "Paleo"

The study of ancestral health is the investigation into how our ancient ancestors lived and what that might tell us about how we can be healthier and happier now. As a field of study, ancestral health (sometimes called "evolutionary health") has been around in some form for hundreds (or arguably thousands) of years—through archeology, paleontology, anthropology, biology, philosophy, and other academic disciplines. Ancestral health scholars have long served up and debated a vast trove of research and theories not just about ancestral diet and movement patterns but also about our forbear's sociocultural patterns, rhythms of life, relational dynamics, belief systems, and so on.[8]

Over the past couple decades, this has become a more popular area of interest and inquiry among nonacademics, too, giving rise to the contemporary "paleo" and "primal" health movements. In just the past few years, a large and growing group of health seekers has enthusiastically embraced ancestrally informed diet and exercise solutions. And for good reason: They tend to work pretty well. One can, without too much disruption, swap a paleo diet for any other diet, or a primal exercise program for any other exercise program, and, if one does it right (eating mostly whole foods and regularly performing a variety of natural, whole-body movements), one can get comparatively good results: Better energy and vitality, lower inflammation, better body-composition, and improved moods and mental focus.

There's no question that ancestrally informed diet and exercise solutions can be helpful, but they can only get us so far. Keep in mind that we live in a culture that *approves* of individuals trying out different diet and exercise programs, particularly if those programs produce weight loss or visually desirable improvements to our physique, and particularly if those programs are media friendly and accompanied by a fleet of specialty products that can be advertised and sold in stores. While your paleo diet or primal workout program might initially seem a little odd to others (those barefoot shoes certainly freaked some people out when they first hit the market), the basic fact that you are *on a diet* or *following a workout program* and that you are *buying a bunch of stuff* to go along with those programs will probably not seem strange in the least.

Unfortunately, beyond diet and exercise, we've been substantially less inclined to focus on the rest of what ancestral health studies have had to teach us. Why is that? Because the other elements of ancient lifestyles are far more complex and intersecting, and as a result, vastly more challenging to integrate into our so-called normal daily lives. *You can't accomplish these changes just by eating different food products or by working out at a different kind of gym.*

The sociocultural and psychospiritual elements of ancestral, tribal, and nomadic life simply don't translate well to our modern way of being. They don't sync up with our economy, our institutions, our social structures, our daily patterns, or seasonal rhythms of life. Consider, for example, these points of difference:

- In our ancestral, hunter-gatherer past, interdependent, collaborative, purpose-centered community was the norm. Whatever you did as an individual directly served and benefitted the people you cared for and relied on. Your efforts, pooled with those of others, directly staved off danger and death and added tangible value to your communal way of life. There was survival-level significance built into just about all your daily endeavors, including small-scale manual tasks. You were guided by elders and were held responsible for the formation of the youth in your tribe. You had a clear sense of purpose, and you were surrounded by others who did too.

- Virtually all work—from finding, gathering, tracking, hunting, and preparing food to fashioning tools, making garments, and building shelters—was collaborative, collective, and multigenerational. People chatted, bonded, and learned from each other while they worked. If you had a problem, everybody knew about it, and everybody wanted to help solve it. Because if you had a problem, it was *the whole tribe's* problem.

- Performing challenging, hands-on tasks with carefully honed skills kept you busy and engaged in creative problem solving and likely produced a series of what we now actively seek out as "flow state" experiences (I'll talk more about psychologist Mihaly Csikszentmihalyi's concept of flow in chapter 4). Those task-based efforts had inherent meaning because they produced communally needed and appreciated outcomes, like nourishment, shelter, tools, garments, and things of utility, significance, and beauty.

- Material surpluses and shortfalls were shared. Significant wealth disparities were essentially unknown. There were not a lot of complicated choices presented to you, no consumer options to consider, little or no social strata to navigate. Everybody lived pretty much the same way and struggled with the same challenges. Your tribe noticed and reflected back to you your greatest areas of natural strength (whether scouting, hunting, gathering, healing, making tools, or mending conflicts) and valued your contributions.

- In ancient tribal reality, there was (we know from archeology and anthropology) an overarching sense of the sacred and a profound connection with nature and with the mysteries of the universe that imbued everyday life. You didn't have to go to church to get your spiritual fix. The natural world abounded in wonder, awe, magic, and mythology. The specific color of the sunrise, the shifting of weather patterns, the appearance of certain plants or animals, the moving constellations in the night sky—these things all had meaning and merited close attention. Sacred rituals and the lessons of ancestral origin stories were infused into everyday routines.

These are not easy things to emulate in the context of modern life. If you tried, people would probably think you had gone crazy, were on drugs, or perhaps had joined a cult. Plus, even if we could easily embrace these changes, we probably wouldn't be inclined to. We've spent tens of thousands of years "improving" on our ancestral past. We've been sold on the idea that this early-era way of life was harder, more dangerous, and less comfortable—or to borrow Thomas Hobbes's words, "nasty, brutish, and short."

But was there really more drudgery and more suffering ten thousand years ago? That's arguable. There was undoubtedly a great deal of difficulty, discomfort, and danger, but it was difficulty, discomfort, and danger of a kind we were then radically more equipped to handle. After all, as a species, we had 2.5 million years to rise to those challenges, to learn those skills, to fine-tune our coping and survival strategies. Science suggests we were pretty successful in that regard. Most experts posit that our ancestors had several *more* hours of leisure time each day than we do (for creative arts, resting, hanging out with loved ones, and so on), not fewer.

Of course, without antibiotics and reliable food supplies, with more opportunities to fall from trees and cliffs, and more predatory animals roaming about, it is true many of our ancestors lived considerably shorter lives than we do. But their shorter lives may well have been more vibrant and gratifying.

A significant body of research shows that depression, loneliness, boredom, and anxiety were (and still are) comparatively rare in traditional hunter-gatherer cultures.[9] In fact, all of the leading causes of death referenced above and listed in endnote 7 (with the possible exception of some deaths by accident)[10] are directly or indirectly tied to what we now call the "diseases of civilization" or "diseases of modernity." According to the World Health Organization, depression is now projected to become the world's leading disease burden by 2030.

I'm not saying that we should (or could) go back to living the way our ancestors did. (I love my flush toilet, and I'm grateful not to have coyotes sniffing around my bed at night.) What I am saying is that when we ignore the programming of our DNA, we do so at our peril. As noted, the field of ancestral health teaches all of this—but to date, what we have heard broadcast most often, seen marketed most aggressively, and been most inclined to incorporate into our daily lives is largely about diet and exercise.

Here's the problem with that: *The challenges we are dealing with now are not limited to diet and exercise.* Rather, they extend to our whole way of being in and relating to the world around us. When we focus obsessively on diet and exercise, though, that's easy for us to miss. So let's take a moment and see what we've been missing.

The Really, Really Big Picture

In chapter 1, I gave you a sense of just how few people are currently healthy, happy, and on track to stay that way. What I didn't explain is that all of that colossal health struggle is set against a backdrop of unprecedented spending.

Here in the United States, beyond the trillions of dollars we are spending within the health-care system, we are spending more than a trillion more on nonmedical health and wellness—from diet aids and fitness interventions to meal delivery, massage, mindfulness, and meditation. And this isn't true just of the United States. According to the Global Wellness Institute, the worldwide wellness industry is now a $4.2 trillion enterprise, and for the past few years, it has been growing at *twice* the rate of the global economy.

In an era when so many of us are demonstrably eager to improve our health, and when we are spending money hand over fist to get healthier, why aren't we having more success? How did we get to a place where our whole way of being in the world doesn't really work for us, and where we repeatedly get hoodwinked into seeing diet and exercise as the cure for all things?

The answer is simple—and yet it can be surprisingly slippery to grasp, in part because it involves ancient history that most of us are never taught to see as relevant to our present-day lives. But it is, so let me give you a quick recap.

Many of our modern-day challenges have their roots in the Agricultural Revolution of about ten thousand years ago. However, to *really* understand our current conundrum, we have to go back a bit farther. Okay, a lot farther—about 2.5 million years—to the dawn of humanity.

Visualized as a timeline, our journey looks kind of like the graph below, except that if the graph were drawn to scale, and the flat part of the timeline wasn't broken, the dot representing the dawn of humanity would be placed about *fifty-two feet further to the left.*

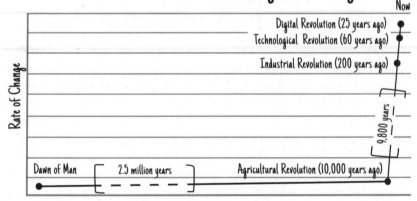

Unprecedented Rate of Social, Environmental and Technological Change

Now

Digital Revolution (25 years ago)
Technological Revolution (60 years ago)

Industrial Revolution (200 years ago)

Rate of Change

9,800 years

Dawn of Man   2.5 million years   Agricultural Revolution (10,000 years ago)

Span of Human Evolution (not to scale)

I didn't think I'd able to convince my publisher to include the hundred extra pages it would have taken to show the fifty-two additional feet required to draw the above graph to scale. So please take a moment now, if you will, and just imagine about one hundred of these pages lined up to your left, flowing across the floor, likely through the wall, perhaps outside the building and down the block. Fifty-two feet of pages, for the record, is about the length of one and a half school busses.

Clearly, I am trying to pack a great deal of history into a very small graph, so let's look at it a different way. If 2.5 million years of human history were shrunk down to the equivalent of a single year, the span of the last ten thousand years (which occupies about a quarter inch in the above graph) would represent just 1.46 days—about thirty-five hours. Relatively speaking, that is not a lot of time. And that's a big part of the problem (problems) we're now facing. Our bodies have no idea how to make sense of the circumstances in which they are enmeshed. The way of life to which they became genetically, metabolically, and neurologically adapted over millions of years, the environments that natural selection prepared them to survive and thrive in—these circumstances are no more.

Our Slow Emergency

As noted, for most of our 2.5 million years, we humans lived as nomadic hunter-gatherers, living communally in small tribes, cobbling together our own makeshift shelters, making our own tools, subsisting on whatever seasonally available plants and animals we could find, and expanding vast quantities of physical energy in the process. Then, over the course of just a few thousand years (a *super* sudden change by evolutionary standards), most humans were thrust into an agrarian world, resulting in rapid and dramatic shifts in our diet, culture, habits, and way of life.

The Agricultural Revolution was the beginning of what turned out to be, for us, a huge leap forward, as well as the beginning of a slow, ten-thousand-year evolutionary emergency. Within the span of a dozen generations, instead of chasing down wild food, we began to grow and store our own. We started developing stockpiles of surplus goods, developing more specialized skills and trading for what we wanted, rather than finding or making things for ourselves. We also started rapidly growing our population, simultaneously expanding and diluting our social connections, living in villages, owning private property and permanent shelters, creating stratified gaps between the haves and have-nots, and reducing our exposure and sense of connection with the natural world.

As our material surpluses and our choices increased, our quest for wealth and social status intensified. We became less cooperative and interdependent with our fellow community members and more inclined to manipulate, abuse, oppress, and enslave them for our benefit. As we became more separated from our natural environment and more isolated from each other, our ways of relating to each other and of finding purpose in our lives shifted dramatically.

That's a shocking amount of change in a relatively short period of time, but it's only the beginning of the evolutionary mismatch our bodies and minds now face. Because about two hundred years ago (using the same relative one-year timeline as above, that's the equivalent of about forty-two minutes), we got smacked with the Industrial Revolution. It brought us all sorts of labor-saving machines, electric lights, urban living, factory jobs, processed foods, mass-produced goods, modern medicine, and printed mass media. It also brought a huge uptick in the use of fossil fuels and the production of toxic pollutants.

Then, soon thereafter (about sixty years ago, the equivalent of about twelve minutes), we got walloped by the Technological Revolution. It delivered all sorts of life-easing, labor-saving automation, plus television, radio, mass-market advertising, and computers. We also got artificial flavors, colors, and lab-created preservatives, mass-produced plastics, nuclear power, nuclear weapons, and a lot more toxic pollutants.

Then, just twenty-five years ago (the equivalent of less than five minutes), we got the Digital Revolution, bringing with it smartphones, social media, screen-based everything, artificial intelligence, drones, Amazon Prime, and still more pollution—as well as a growing awareness that our activities are driving widespread ecosystem destruction and climate change that could soon render the earth uninhabitable by us and a lot of other creatures.[11]

That means for 99.99 percent of human history we lived more or less one way: active, subsistence focused, eating whole foods, observing natural daily rhythms of light and dark, spending a significant amount of time in the unpolluted outdoors, surrounded by a small tribe of deeply connected, interdependent people who saw the sacred in everyday life, who saw nature as the source of all things, and literally worshipped the ground they walked on. And then, boom, pretty much everything changed.

Today, we're mostly sedentary, simultaneously overfed and undernourished by mechanically processed foods, and separated from natural rhythms. We spend most of our time indoors or in polluted outdoor environments, surrounded by electronics and consumer products, continuously bombarded by mass media, chronically stressed, materially focused, and with limited time, attention, and energy to invest in meaningful relationships or supportive social connections. And we live in existential dread about the potential for the end of the world as we know it. Meanwhile, almost nothing within our basic biological or operational systems has kept pace with this rapid cultural and environmental change.

Our Evolutionary Mismatch

Several thousand years (or even a few hundred years) might sound like a lot, but it's simply not enough time to have permitted our DNA—the genetic instructions that dictate how our bodies develop, function, and respond—to adjust very much. All of this has given rise to the nasty condition known as "evolutionary mismatch."

Evolutionary mismatch is what happens when you take an organism that has spent 2.5 million years of physiological adaptation and trait development preparing for one set of conditions, and you abruptly thrust that organism into a set of circumstances for which it is entirely unprepared. What you end up with is a weird and rather desperate set of maladaptations, the kind that negatively affect virtually every system in that organism's body-mind. In this case, that organism is you. It's me. It's all of us. So, it's absolutely critical to remember this:

> ## We are the first generation of humans ever to have been exposed to anything remotely like our current circumstances.

We are, in effect, an unprecedented living experiment. The scope and intensity of evolutionary mismatch we're dealing with now is historically unparalleled. The disconnect between our genetic programming and our current way of life is so extreme, so pervasive, and so destructive that it really can't be ignored. Yet ignore it we do.

For the sake of our health, our sanity, and our survival, we have to stop doing that. But how? I've found it helps to give the largely invisible, intangible, yet incontrovertible context of our modern-day existence a name. I call it the Unhealthy Default Reality (or sometimes, for short, the UDR).

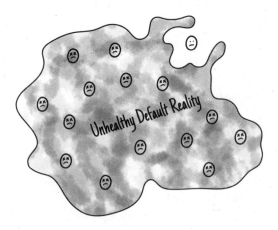

Understanding the Unhealthy Default Reality

The Unhealthy Default Reality is the combined result of our evolutionary mismatch and our mass-culture reaction to it. It is both the ragged wound formed when we were torn from our hunter-gatherer roots and the messy layers of bandages, ointments, and magic-bullet cures we've heaped on top of that wound in an effort to cope. It's depression *and* pharmaceutical antidepressants. It's obesity *and* the bikini-body-obsessed weight-loss industry. It's the rash *and* the anti-itch cream. It's dark circles *and* 260 kinds of under-eye concealer. It's the constant, inescapable barrage of noise *and* the fact that so many people are now wearing headphones to avoid it.

> The Unhealthy Default Reality is, in effect, "the crazy that passes for normal."

It's the unprecedented, discordant, inherently stressful, and often alienating nature of our present-day social, cultural, environmental milieu. Defined by accelerating change, speed, complexity, and uncertainty, the Unhealthy Default Reality is always operating in the background of our daily experiences and assumptions. It is the foundation of our existence, the stage on which all actions and transactions take place. It occupies the spaces between us and our daily choices, in the connections between us and everyone to whom we relate.

The Unhealthy Default Reality is the predominant context in which we now live. Or try to, anyway. A lot of us recognize that we are suffering at the hands of the Unhealthy Default Reality, and we see others around us suffering, but we don't fully comprehend why. For the most part, we don't question it. We don't talk about it much. We're too busy just trying to survive.

When we're fully embedded within the Unhealthy Default Reality, and when our daily lives, choices and perspectives are largely dictated by it, it's not something we can easily see or hold in our conscious awareness. We have too much of our attention focused on problems that *seem* more pressing. And *that,* my friends, is how the Unhealthy Default Reality keeps us in its grip.

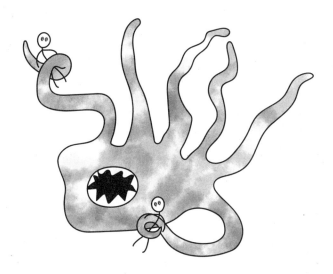

Why the Unhealthy Default Reality Is Hard to See

The Unhealthy Default Reality is a consummate shape-shifter and illusionist. One of its favorite tricks involves a classic "can't see the forest for the trees" scenario. We are all kept so busy struggling with our own individual health-threatening "trees"—things like weight gain, fatigue, illness, stress, depression, anxiety, loneliness, and feelings of inadequacy—that we remain largely oblivious to the broader societal and environmental "forest" in which those widely shared problems are firmly rooted. We fail to see the substrate in which all our personal problems are planted and by which they are perennially sustained and encouraged to grow.

Seeing our health challenges through this larger "forest" lens can transform the way we relate to them. It can help us get enough depersonalized distance to go about addressing those challenges more strategically. But that shift toward a broader and deeper perspective isn't something that comes naturally to most of us. There are many reasons for this. Let's take a look at just a few of them.

EDUCATION

First, the scope of natural and human history is not something most Americans are taught as children—by our families or in school. We might learn a little dominant-culture-filtered history (for example, some sanitized version of how Western pioneer settlers or early Native Americans supposedly lived), but we generally don't study much in the way of anthropology or sociology, at least until college. We aren't taught to connect the dots between most of the subjects we study, much less connect them to our own and others' lives.

Even after we become adults, most of us simply aren't encouraged or trained to look at our own place in nature or our current culture (much less others' cultures) in an objective, historically contextual or critical way. We're not predisposed to think in terms of intersecting community, environment, or societal challenges. On the contrary, we're taught to concern ourselves primarily with our own individual interests, our personal desires, our seemingly unique pain-points in the context of the right-here-and-now. What we're taught to focus on, in other words, is a bunch of seemingly unrelated trees.

MEDIA

Next, the broad-and-deep is not a perspective to which the popular media is inclined to give much coverage. Again, there are a number of reasons for this. Research consistently shows that as contemporary media consumers, most of us are not particularly interested in pondering deep, complex, and potentially murky subjects. We're far more attracted to the media equivalent of bright, shiny objects: Fun, easy, sensational pieces about celebrities and makeovers; brief, bulleted lists; breezy how-to content focused on incrementally improving this or that aspect of our body, romantic life, finances, fashion sense, and so on.

We've been trained by our media experience not only to accept this sort of superficiality but also to expect and demand more of the same. As a result, the media content we consume on a daily basis is simultaneously being designed around our ever-shortening attention spans *and further exacerbating them.* Video gets sliced into tinier and tinier segments. Sound bytes are doled out in syllables and abbreviated character sets rather than words, sentences, and paragraphs. Meanwhile, the "solutions" we're presented with become increasingly simplistic, prescriptive, and superficial. As one book agent told me (by way of explaining why this book would never sell): *People don't want vitamins; they want pain pills.*

Of course, popular media hasn't been designed just around *our* preferences. Advertisers and sponsors, too, are enthusiastic about supporting light, airy, sensational content that drives consumer desires. They have a lot of pain pills to sell, so when placing ads, they overwhelmingly seek out (and thus fiscally support) media that proposes an ample supply of consumer-oriented solutions. Understandably, most advertisers would prefer to be associated with gear guides, celebrity profiles, product reviews, and "listicles" (5 Simple Weight-Loss Secrets!) than have their ads sitting alongside complex, ponderous, and potentially disturbing articles about social, cultural, environmental, and historical concerns that they suspect (rightly) almost nobody will read.[12]

This means a lot of the deeper, more contextualized, and significant information (the kind of information we need to make sense of our world) simply never gets published or aired in compelling ways. And when it does, it is not aggressively promoted. It doesn't "click" well, in digital-media speak, and so it never gets elevated above the fold or moved to the front page of whatever website or app you're browsing. It doesn't take long before deeper, more probing articles are buried by celebrity weight-loss tips that click much better. And the fact that those celebrity weight-loss tips click better means that publishers can now point to hard data *definitively proving* that this sort of material is what their audience *really* wants to see.

INDUSTRY AND GOVERNMENT

Perhaps even more distressing than the in-your-face influences that undermine the quality of health-related information you see are the hidden influences that most of us never see at all. Cozy industry ties and aggressive corporate propaganda campaigns influence scientific research, suppress negative media stories, and sneakily influence everything from the USDA Nutrition Guidelines to public health policies.

We got a distressing example of the latter in February 2019 when a news story that should have provoked public outrage and a congressional inquiry instead landed with little more than a thud and a yawn. Salon.com reported it this way:[13]

> *A paper published this week, which analyzed private emails exchanged between the Centers for Disease Control and Prevention (CDC) and Coca-Cola, revealed that the sugary drink corporation has for years been a secret voice of influence on the public health policy decisions of a US federal agency that is supposed to protect Americans' health. The private emails speak of a federal agency hopelessly corrupted by a powerful corporation that has squirreled its way into the public dialogue on health and intentionally obfuscated scientific studies and narratives that threatened their profit margins.*

So, there's all that,[14] and then there's another (and somewhat related) influencing factor: The constricted, myopic lens of our health-care system.

CONVENTIONAL MEDICINE

First, let me say that I do not intend to bash doctors and nurses here—they are some of the hardest-working and best-intentioned people I know. It must simply be acknowledged that the nature and basis of our collective suffering is not something the conventional medical system is remotely prepared to address.[15]

We've been trained to look to doctors for health advice. We take their diagnoses, their views of cause and cure as reality. But today's doctors were never trained to make sense of the health problems we are now facing. In medical school, they get only few hours of nutrition education (much of it ill founded and outdated), and they spend far more time learning how to diagnose rare disorders and infectious diseases than they do learning to wrestle with the most pervasive body-mind miseries that the majority of us are suffering. Many have also gotten a lot of their training directly from pharmaceutical companies (notorious for influencing not just individual providers' health counsel but also public health policy).[16]

Let's face it, most of our medical professionals are struggling with health problems themselves. The majority of them have very little idea how our common, complex, and chronic disease states can be constructively addressed through lifestyle adjustments—particularly in the context of a culture that makes those lifestyle adjustments woefully difficult. Additionally, even if our conventionally trained medical professionals *did* have the training and background to effectively address the root causes of chronic disease, in the context of our current health-care system, they would probably not be much help. Currently, there's no time (and no incentive) for most doctors to walk their patients through a thorough analysis of their health problems, much less present thoughtful, personalized, realistic solutions to the socially and environmentally entrenched challenges those patients are facing.

The overburdened primary-care model mostly revolves around ten-minute appointments, easy-access symptom-suppressing prescriptions, and insurance-reimbursable fee-for-service medical procedures. These appointments are eventually followed up with referrals to specialists for the increasingly complex problems that predictably proceed from this ineffective approach. Throughout our conventional health-care system, the focus is not on healing or health, it is on compliance with disease-management and symptom-treatment programs. It has become, as many progressive health experts and advocates have noted, more of a sick-care system.

Even so-called preventative medicine is now mostly focused on things like vaccinations, cancer screenings, and "knowing your numbers." These programs are good at telling patients the obvious (that they are overweight and at risk for illness, for example) and good at funneling them into early-treatment programs (including, perhaps, counterproductive diet and exercise programs), but they almost never dig into the meaty topics most essential to the actual prevention of common chronic diseases. And to be fair, many patients aren't particularly open to hearing that resolving their health ailments will require significantly changing their daily lives. Which brings us to …

US

Because our Unhealthy Default Reality is not a pleasant thing to consider, and not something we're are encouraged by our families, educators, media, or medical experts to individually investigate or challenge, it's not something we are inclined to collectively acknowledge or to openly discuss with each other. Instead, we stay focused on our stressful personal problems of the moment. We either try to follow the treatments, programs, and interventions we are prescribed, or we push our health problems to the periphery of our awareness as best we can, and for as long as we can, we muddle through.

As a result, the greatest threats to our well-being operate "out of sight, out of mind"—even when they are right there, dictating our decisions, aggressively undermining our health and happiness in real time. In effect, by submitting to this state of affairs, we unwittingly help create, condone, and sustain the circumstances of our oppression.

Choosing to be a healthy person in an unhealthy world means taking on the role of an intentional outlier. It means walking against the traffic of a mass hallucination a lot of the time. That's not something most people are prepared for, and therein lies the rub:

The real problem is not just that making healthy change is difficult in our culture. It's that it's difficult for reasons that are not openly acknowledged, much less effectively addressed.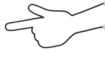

The good news is that we can change that. We just need to begin seeing and talking more about what's really happening to us and about the fact that this is a pervasive and shared—not rare or individual—experience.

Getting a Clearer View

I know, I've given you a lot to think about. By now, you might be wondering if it's even possible to overcome all the forces that are working against you. Trust me, it is. But seeing the Unhealthy Default Reality for what it is takes both initiative and guts. It is not something you can do casually or half-heartedly. On the contrary, it requires going down the sort of rabbit hole Morpheus presented to Neo in *The Matrix*. And that requires willingly pulling your attention away from a thousand more immediate and seemingly important problems that the Unhealthy Default Reality throws in your face daily, thereby blocking your view of just about everything else. The next two illustrations reflect what we see and are culturally encouraged to deal with—and what we are typically convinced to overlook or ignore.

Figure 1

What We Are Encouraged to See

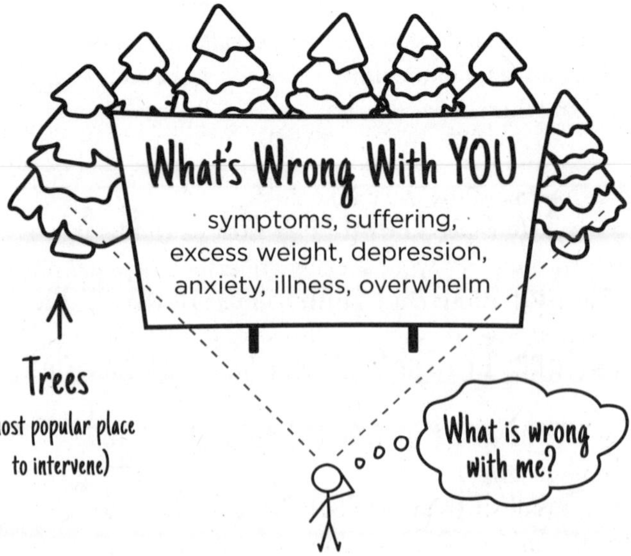

What's Wrong With YOU
symptoms, suffering, excess weight, depression, anxiety, illness, overwhelm

Trees
(most popular place to intervene)

What is wrong with me?

Figure 2

What We Can See When We Step Out of Line ...

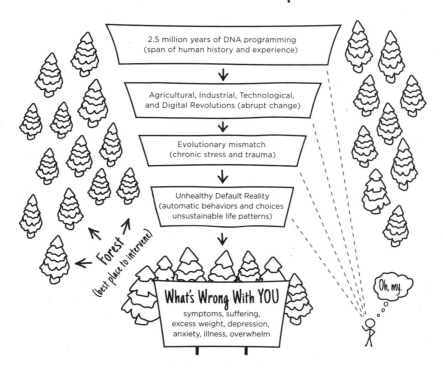

Figure 1 represents the tree-level version of reality that we are encouraged to see by our mass culture. This is what we are urged to keep our attention and resources trained on, typically to the exclusion of all else. This is life according to the Unhealthy Default Reality.

Figure 2 shows a bigger and very different view. This is what it is *possible* to see when you step out of your socially prescribed "normal" position and when you refuse to be limited by the problem-solution strictures of the Unhealthy Default Reality. The top two boxes of figure 2 represent everything that occurred in that 2.5-million-year timeline chart I showed you earlier in this chapter—and all of the unprecedented social, environmental, and technical changes that humans have experienced as a result. The third box represents the resulting evolutionary mismatch we are living with now, as well as all the chronic stresses and recurring traumas that mismatch brings to bear. The fourth box represents the domain of the Unhealthy Default Reality and our tacit, unconscious acceptance of its dominant viewpoints, automatic behaviors, and preprogrammed choices. The final box (the only one we can typically see, as in figure 1, because it is pushed right up against our faces) represents the predictable outcomes of our current condition, namely a wide array of symptoms, suffering, and ongoing degradations of our body-mind.

The first and second boxes of figure 2 would be wise things for us to take stock of, because seeing and understanding these things more clearly would help us find more compassion for ourselves and others. It would help us see how we could get into greater agreement with our shared history and genetic programming and into better alignment with the natural world around us. The third and fourth boxes, meanwhile, are probably the best, most effective places for us to intervene and make adjustments on a daily basis.

But that's not what the Unhealthy Default Reality encourages us to do. Instead, it throws up that giant, horizon-blocking billboard emblazoned with a rotating gallery of "What Is Wrong with *You*" messages, which effectively keeps us from seeing anything else. And so we remain intently focused on our litany of "personal" health and fitness problems and largely ignorant (or at least functionally unaware) of the universally experienced circumstances from which those problems sprang.

This is one of Unhealthy Default Reality's most ingenious schemes. While you are busy obsessing about *your* weight issue, *your* rash, *your* indigestion, *your* depression or anxiety or perceived inadequacy, the Unhealthy Default Reality is cranking out a whole slew of "solutions" to your problems. Mostly, these are solutions that require you to hand over large sums of money to large corporations for the rest of your life.

This arrangement has not been working out very well for most of us. But it has been growing our economy at an impressive clip. Because, in the wise words of Wendell Berry, "What's wrong with us generates more GNP than what's right with us." Translation: The more we can be convinced we are inherently lacking or inadequate, the more we can be convinced to buy—and the more easily we can be sold.

Stepping Out of Line

So how can we see beyond the Unhealthy Default Reality's trees and start dealing with the more significant forest in our midst? Taking a Healthy Deviant view involves taking just a few bold steps to one side, pulling ourselves away from the "what's wrong with us" billboard to get a better vantage point on the conditions that are giving us trouble. Seeing things from this deeper and more wide-angled view empowers us to strategically adjust our lives in ways that:

- Prepare us to better perceive our Unhealthy Default Reality at work.

- Strengthen our ability to minimize or avoid the negative impacts of its destructive norms and influences, including default, automatic behaviors and choices.

- Cease wasting our time, attention, energy, money, and other resources on distractions and largely ineffective symptom-level interventions.

- Participate in a larger movement that helps to positively evolve our circumstances and our collective responses to them over time.

While addressing the domain of our current shared condition is of prime importance, there's nothing inherently wrong with *also* acknowledging and directly addressing our personal symptoms (excess weight, illness, anxiety, etc.). There's nothing wrong with *also* adjusting the way we eat and move in ways that feel good to us. In fact, for those who can successfully manage them, programmatic interventions at the level of diet and exercise can be profoundly empowering, leading naturally to subsequent steps in decoupling from the Unhealthy Default Reality. (More on those soon.) But for many people, making prescribed changes to diet and exercise either proves maddeningly impossible or insanely confusing—or it requires so much body-mind bandwidth that it torpedoes any other meaningful efforts toward healthy change.

If we tackle our symptoms without a deeper understanding of the context that's producing those symptoms, we don't stand much of a chance of developing the awareness, motivation, and skills required to shift our circumstances. We have very little opportunity to sustainably change our automatic, default behaviors in a positive direction, and until we do that, we are destined to remain both victims and perpetuators of the Unhealthy Default Reality. Despite our best intentions, we will naturally find ourselves reverting to the default choices and experiences our society presents as "normal," then struggling to correct the inevitable, multiplying outcomes. We'll be feeding quarters into a whack-a-mole game we can never win—attacking one set of symptoms only to find another set popping up in its place.

Whack-a-Symptom Game

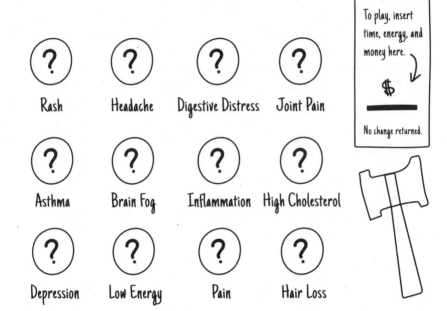

Distracted, depleted—bamboozled into complacent suffering and compulsive "problem-solving"—we will never recognize the true costs doing business with the Unhealthy Default Reality on its terms, or the range of better options available to us. Even if we manage to deal with our most vexing symptoms of the moment (dropping the excess weight, clearing the rash, taming our runaway anxiety), we will do so at an outsized monetary and energetic expense. We'll be dealing with the trees, not the forest. And the forest will forever be producing more trees.

That's why I'm making a case for abandoning our assigned tree-and-branch-inspecting position and taking up a new lookout with a much better view of the entire forest. This view may look and feel a little weird at first. It represents a very powerful and socially unsanctioned perspective shift. And it may not be one your friends, family, or boss will share, understand or in any way approve of. It will probably not be a viewpoint you'll see morning talk show hosts advance, that you'll see advertisements support, or that your doctor will make time to discuss with you (except, perhaps, in the event he or she refers you to a psychiatrist for further evaluation). It's probably not what the futurists at the Davos World Economic Forum are going to be excitedly hailing as the next big thing. Why? Because it's hard to sell a lot of solutions to people who don't perceive themselves as having a lot of problems.

This is part of why looking—*really* looking—at the Unhealthy Default Reality is such a revolutionary act. It throws a lot of assumptions into question, and it throws a lot of our consumer behavior into disarray. If we stop buying the solutions the Unhealthy Default Reality presents as necessary for fixing all we see as "wrong with us," a lot of our economy would radically shift. But once you start seeing things from this clearer vantage point, and once you begin to connect with others who are seeing the same things you do, life gets easier. Health improvement becomes easier, and also more fun. Because once you recognize our Unhealthy Default Reality—and its agenda for you and everybody you know—you have already taken a huge, game-changing step toward freeing yourself from its grip.

Feeling a little looser in your societal straightjacket? Excellent. The next step involves seeing how the Unhealthy Default Reality has been turning your own self-improvement efforts against you. And how you can stop it.

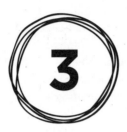

The Misunderstood Problem

The significant problems we have cannot be solved at the
same level of thinking with which we created them.

—ALBERT EINSTEIN

In chapter 2, I described the nature of our evolutionary mismatch, and I explained how the Unhealthy Default Reality that emerged from that mismatch has been increasingly messing with our health and happiness. I also explained why it's often difficult to see the machinations of the Unhealthy Default Reality at work. Now I want to help you get even clearer about one of the Unhealthy Default Reality's most brilliant strategies for camouflaging itself and covering its tracks: *It simply insists that our health problems are entirely of our own making.*

Here's the story the Unhealthy Default Reality tells:

No matter how many unhealthy things the marketplace presents us with …

No matter how appealing advertising makes them seem …

No matter how pervasive unhealthy choices are in our environment …

No matter how much damage unhealthy products do to our collective health …

No matter how much unhealthy products are incentivized and subsidized at taxpayer expense …

No matter how huge the institutional barriers and health disparities …

It is always entirely up to each of us to manage our health choices all on our own, to decide precisely how much unhealthy stuff we allow into our bodies, and to overcome all obstacles to living a healthy lifestyle.

Industry front groups like the Center for Consumer Freedom (an organization that has spent millions promoting unfettered, unregulated access to things like cigarettes, fast food, and candy) are especially fond of insisting on this idea. They like to argue that everything is fine in moderation (even when those things have been purposefully designed to be addictive) that virtually anything (including the most inflammation-producing things imaginable) "can be part of healthy lifestyle," and that each of us is personally responsible for making "good choices." Oh, and we just need to be more "active."

In theory, it is true that it is ultimately up to us to decide what goes into our bodies. But practically speaking, it is also true that the Unhealthy Default Reality (UDR) both radically limits our available choices and aggressively undermines our ability to make sensible decisions (for more on that, see "The Ape in the Arcade" later in this chapter). The circumstances and available options within our neighborhoods, schools, workplaces, health-care environments, places of worship, and recreation centers are all massively influenced by the downstream effects of the mindsets, policies, and prescribed preferences of the UDR. The media amplifies and promotes the prescribed preferences of the UDR in almost everything it does.

So while healthy choices and moderation are both great things to celebrate, it's not like making healthy, moderate choices is something we do on a level playing field. Unhealthy choices are constantly foisted upon us, modeled for us, dangled in front of us, and incentivized for us, while healthy choices require a prohibitive amount of effort, ingenuity, and expense. In short, our entire society is wired to get us to want, buy, consume, and do the things that reliably break us down.

While we are at it, let's also acknowledge the painfully obvious truth that healthy choices are a whole lot easier for some of us than for others. The less money and education we have, the more aggressively we are discriminated against (on the basis of race, ethnicity, gender, sexual orientation, age, etc.), and the fewer supportive systems we have in place, the more difficult, stressful, and dangerous our lives tend to become; the more likely we are to be targeted by vulture-like industries; and the less likely we will be to access easily (much less afford) "healthy choices" on a daily basis.

Even for those of us who aren't struggling with overt discrimination, in the context of the UDR, making a single healthy choice can cost us so much—in terms of effort, energy, time, money, and focus (as well as social discomfort)—that it puts the next healthy choice even further out of reach. To counteract these challenges, we must keep reminding ourselves and each other that the primary problem is not that we are inadequate, flawed, or inherently weak willed. The problem is that we are too oppressed by the Unhealthy Default Reality to break free from it.

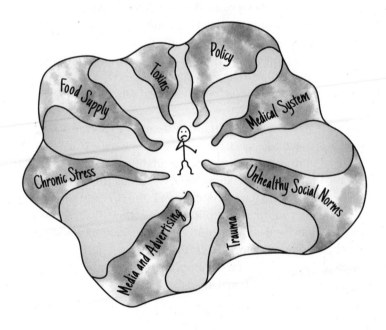

The Unhealthy Default Reality at Work

"The hardest thing to explain," philosopher Ayn Rand once wrote, "is the glaringly evident which everybody has decided not to see." Well, here's one such glaringly evident problem: We are all too worn out, freaked out, or brain addled to put up much of a fight against the forces that are making us ill.

A great many of those forces hide out, often in plain sight, within a system I call the vicious cycle of the Unhealthy Default Reality.

Vicious Cycle of the Unhealthy Default Reality

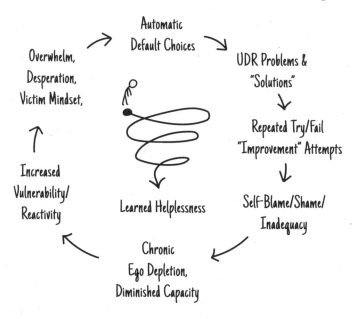

It works something like this:

- The Unhealthy Default Reality presents us with a version of "normal" life that makes unhealthy patterns, attitudes, and choices easy, automatic, seemingly cheap, and socially acceptable (while also making healthy choices difficult, inconvenient, comparatively expensive, and weird).

- We adopt the unhealthy default patterns and choices (conventional ideals, nutrient-poor processed foods, sedentary work and play, inadequate sleep, weak social connections, passive consumption of media, little to no time in nature, etc.).

- We get inflamed, sick, heavy, depressed, anxious, and insecure.

- The Unhealthy Default Reality points out that we are not living up to accepted standards and serves up diets, exercise programs, consumer goods, miracle cures, self-help strategies, and medical interventions that promise to solve, ameliorate, or camouflage our perceived problems.

- We expend huge resources (time, effort, money, willpower) on these things, but we find they mostly don't work as promised, and/or that we cannot practically integrate them into our lives, or that they have undesirable side effects.

- Finding ourselves still not good enough (and perhaps now wrong in *new* ways) we blame ourselves and become convinced that we are weak willed and undisciplined, or simply unfixable.

- We don't want others to know about our failings or inadequacy. We decide to just try harder.

- We expend more resources on more solutions, which also don't work for us. We begin employing more self-numbing and self-distracting strategies (drugs, alcohol, video games, media, shopping, social media, casual sex, etc.)

- Our resources and vitality are further depleted. We feel even worse about ourselves, so we embrace a variety of unhealthy coping and comfort-seeking strategies, and we become more inflamed, heavy, anxious, and depressed.

- We develop chronic, inflammatory health conditions and eventually receive one or more medical diagnoses that become a central part of our identity.

- We either don't want others to know we are suffering (because this means we are flawed), or we talk a lot about our medically diagnosed diseases by way of explaining why our lives and bodies are the way they are.

- We are encouraged to invest a lot of resources in "treating" (i.e., suppressing the symptoms of) our health conditions.

- The root causes of our health conditions (living within the prescribed rules and patterns of the Unhealthy Default Reality, following the wrongheaded or otherwise unhelpful health advice it doles out) are not acknowledged or effectively addressed by the conventional medical system, the mass media, or most of the people we know (many of whom are suffering from similar conditions).

- As we become more chronically depleted and inflamed, we become more desperate, less capable of coping with our lives, and more vulnerable to the Unhealthy Default Reality's next socially promoted solution, intervention, or distraction.

- We may become increasingly hopeless, helpless, and apathetic, or we may go into fix-it overdrive, becoming zealously devoted to strict diet and exercise solutions that keep our symptoms at bay. In this case, we may present ourselves as being healthier and happier than we really are, perhaps telling others how to fix themselves by doing what we are doing, even though we are feeling increasingly panicked or dead inside. A huge amount of our life force is expended in trying to do all the right things, be all the right things, to sell other people on solutions, and to appear successful at all costs.

- This depleting cycle of ineffective resource expenditures, reduced resiliency, and lowered self-regard repeats itself until we are husks of our former selves, siphoned of both our internal and external resources, and so firmly under the sway of the Unhealthy Default Reality that we don't recognize there is any other way to be.

- Eventually, we go partially or totally unconscious, losing our sense of dignity, purpose, and potential. Accepting a drastically reduced state of capacity and vitality, we forsake our self-authorship, freedom, and autonomy. We may become desperate or parasitically reliant on others for our survival.

- Meanwhile, this state of decline is also happening to most of the other people we know. It is statistically common. It seems, you know (shrug), *normal.*

- In accepting this regrettable state of affairs as "just the way it is," we become co-opted and assimilated by the Unhealthy Default Reality, thereby expanding its powers and its reach.

Most of us have seen a lot of this playing out in our own lives and the lives of those we love. So, what can we do about it? First, we have to free our minds from the "fix me" ruts in which the Unhealthy Default Reality has programmed them to think.

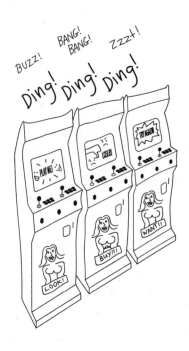

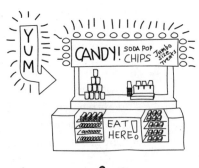

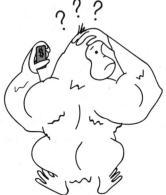

The Ape in the Arcade

We know that environment drives behavior. So what would happen if you were to pull a gorilla out of the wild and plop him into a video-game arcade? How would he likely react to all those crazy lights flashing and all those bells and buzzers going off all around him? What if you were to deprive him of access to natural daylight and natural darkness? What if you gave him access to a fast-food concession stand and candy-filled vending machines as his only source of food and then gave him a debit card to pay for it? What if you gave him access to a device that dispensed arcade tokens—and opioid painkillers?

With no trees to swing on, no plant-covered ground to scratch at for yummy grubs and tubers, and no fellow apes to hang with, how long would this creature likely survive? How would he suffer? How long would it take him to figure out the ATM and learn to play all those arcade games? How long would it take

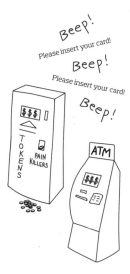

Beep!
Please insert your card!

Beep!
Please insert your card!

Beep!

him to overdose on popcorn or painkillers? By what means would this poor beast likely seek to cope, adapt, or escape before he perished?

Obviously, this would be a disastrous and cruel experiment to run on any living creature. And yet, in many ways, it is akin to the experiment we're currently running on ourselves. Relative to our genetic programming, these are the same kinds of discordant conditions we are challenged to make sense of, adjust to, and find a way to thrive in each and every day of our lives.

Thanks to 2.5 million years of evolution, our DNA is still much more adapted to the natural environments and lifestyles of our simian brethren than it is to the modern mass-culture contexts in which we currently live. Slowly but surely, millennium by millennium, we've been solving some important survival-level problems for ourselves, and in the process, we've been creating many others.

Like that ape in the arcade, we're struggling to cope. We're trying to improvise within the rapidly shifting environments we're creating for ourselves, but a lot of what we are being asked to do doesn't come naturally to us. A lot of our basic needs are not being met in our modern environments and patterns. A lot of the prescribed solutions and easily accessible options we're being presented with are not only working poorly, they are actively working against us.

In many ways, Healthy Deviance is about seeing our challenge as breaking out of the arcade (or radically redesigning it to minimize the evident mismatch) rather than merely trying to subsist there or, worse, scrounging for tokens and trying to beat the high score on whatever arcade game we happen to be playing at the moment.

A New Level of Thinking

Albert Einstein was right when he observed that "the significant problems we have cannot be solved at the same level of thinking with which we created them." And yet that is precisely what millions of health seekers have long been attempting to do, with little or no success. We've been trying to lose weight, battle depression, and "solve" our chronic disease problems using the same quick-fix, short-view, connection-denying mindsets that produced those problems in the first place. This approach has kept us trapped in the UDR, while steadily reinforcing its hold on us.

When you look at it objectively, it's actually a pretty slick system:

1. We are conditioned to unconsciously accept **Unhealthy Default Perspectives** (our society's socially condoned beliefs, assumptions, values, preferences, priorities, and ideals).

2. These perspectives set us up to live in ways that produce **Unhealthy Default Problems** (stress, obesity, inflammatory disease, depression, anxiety, overwork, time poverty, debt, and feelings of inadequacy).

3. Our problems drive us to embrace **Unhealthy Default Solutions** (symptom-suppressing drugs, surgeries, miracle cures, fussy and extreme diet and exercise programs, camouflaging beauty products, self-medication, distraction, and technological devices).

4. These "solutions" rarely resolve the root causes of our complaints, but they do incline us to spend more money (remember the whack-a-mole game?), suffer more stress, and become more desperate, thereby setting us up for more Unhealthy Default Perspectives (self-comparison with unachievable ideals, self-loathing as the result of our perceived failures) as well as more Unhealthy Default Problems (addictions, crises, traumas, unhealthy risk-taking, passivity, financial and legal troubles).

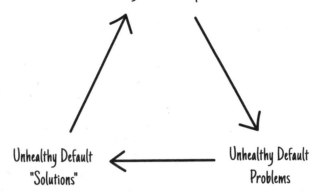

Unhealthy Default Perspectives

Unhealthy Default "Solutions"

Unhealthy Default Problems

With each turn of the cycle, those Unhealthy Default Perspectives, Problems, and Solutions become self-perpetuating. Meanwhile, by virtue of our daily actions and choices, we are unconsciously contributing to, underwriting, and reinforcing the Unhealthy Default Reality, and spreading Unhealthy Default Perspectives around to our friends, families, and coworkers.

The only way to stop doing this is to arrest and reverse this cycle. This starts with recognizing an Unhealthy Default Perspective when you see one. Here is a running list of Unhealthy Default Perspectives that circulate around us almost everywhere we go, particularly as we strive to better ourselves and our lives:

- *New is better.*

- *Faster is better.*

- *Bigger is better.*

- *More is better.*

- *Cheaper is better (except when it's a luxury, indulgent, or "exclusive" product; then expensive is better).*

- *You'd be happier if you were more attractive.*

- *You'd be happier if you had all the right things.*

- *You'd be happier if you were rich and famous.*

- *Celebrities and rich people are happier than you.*

- *Celebrities and rich people are better than you.*

- *The opinions and ideas of celebrities and rich people count more.*
- *Never stop comparing yourself to others, especially celebrities and rich people.*
- *You have to fit in (but still be better than everyone else).*
- *Some body types are better than others.*
- *Some skin, hair, and facial features are better than others.*
- *There are a lot of things wrong with you and your body.*
- *Money can fix most of the things wrong with you.*
- *You should be worried and ashamed about what's wrong with you.*
- *You should fix your visible flaws or hide them—quick.*
- *You might have a disease—you should get a diagnosis.*
- *You are definitely at risk for disease.*
- *We can't really know what causes your disease.*
- *Your disease can't be cured, but it must be treated.*
- *You just need to* manage *your disease.*
- *Focus on suppressing your symptoms.*
- *Pain is the enemy; dull it or numb it any way you can.*
- *When it gets worse, see a specialist.*
- *Diet and exercise might help, but they probably won't be enough.*
- *Eat less, exercise more.*
- *Calories make you fat.*
- *Carbs make you fat.*
- *Fat makes you fat.*
- *Keep track of everything you eat.*
- *Count all the numbers associated with everything you eat.*
- *You must follow this diet exactly.*
- *If that diet doesn't work, try this one.*
- *What you're eating has nothing to do with it.*

- *You should be able to eat however you want.*
- *It's just your genetics.*
- *Keep living the way you always have.*
- *You are eating/exercising/living all wrong.*
- *Science will solve it.*
- *A drug, device, or procedure will solve it.*
- *A home-delivery or subscription service will solve it.*
- *Famous experts and authority figures will tell you how to solve it.*
- *A diet or workout program will solve it.*
- *An app will solve it.*
- *A charm bracelet or affirmation necklace will solve it.*
- *Quick, easy fixes that you can buy are best.*
- *Pay attention to the science.*
- *Don't believe the science.*
- *You can't understand the science.*
- *You're not looking at the right science.*
- *Only scientists can understand science.*
- *Only medical doctors can give health advice.*
- *You are listening to the wrong medical doctors.*
- *Only authority figures know how things work.*
- *You are listening to the wrong authority figures.*
- *Don't make thing so complicated.*
- *You are oversimplifying things.*
- *Keep looking for more and better fixes.*
- *Look for the seal of approval.*
- *You could do better.*
- *You deserve better.*

- *You can have it all, do it all.*
- *You just need to work harder, try harder, do more things, get more things, fix more things.*
- *You are only as good as what you've recently acquired, fixed, and achieved.*
- *Everybody is looking at you, assessing you, judging you, all the time.*
- *Look to the media to tell you what you should be doing and caring about.*
- *See these people in the advertisements? That's what you should be doing/having/being.*
- *You really should be able to do this; it's not that hard.*
- *All the people in the ads and stock photos seem to be doing fine.*
- *Look—healthy living is fun and easy and carefree!*
- *Look—eating salads alone is a delight!*
- *Look—healthy people are perfect and have it all figured out!*
- *A lot of people are doing better than you.*
- *You're not measuring up or fitting in.*
- *Being healthy is a* choice, *so you must be making the wrong choices.*
- *If you can't eat/exercise/live right, it's because you are stupid, inherently lazy, or otherwise flawed.*
- *You need to work on yourself harder.*
- *You really just need more willpower.*

Where Willpower Gets Ugly

Ah yes, willpower. One overarching mindset the UDR teaches is that willpower is the answer to everything. There is a lot of convincing science suggesting that willpower (or rather, *what we think of* as willpower) really is a big factor in determining life outcomes, including the trajectory of our health, career, finances, relationships, and more. But here's what most Healthy Deviants have learned the hard way:

What looks like a problem of insufficient willpower is often a problem of chronic depletion and distraction.

And guess what? Chronic depletion and distraction are the natural by-products of the unholy alliance between our Unhealthy Default Reality and the opportunistic "health improvement" industries it has spawned.

This is a diabolical sort of double whammy, and it operates much like Munchausen syndrome by proxy. The Unhealthy Default Reality first induces our illness and/or convinces us of our inadequacy. Then it foists a variety of "care" and "improvement" interventions upon us in ways that further undermine our autonomy and degrade our well-being.

Let me be clear about this: It's not just that many of the most broadly promoted and profitable health "solutions" don't help very much; it's that *they very often make things worse,* further precipitating the downward spiral the Unhealthy Default Reality put into motion. By putting immense drains on our vitality and resources, the most common, conventional health-care and health-improvement solutions have steadily made us sicker, fatter, more vulnerable, more ashamed, and more inclined to just give up.

Take conventional dietary advice, for example. For decades, we've been getting terrible, industry-influenced dietary counsel from the USDA via their nutritional guidelines, food pyramid, and MyPlate.gov. Rather than curbing the expansion of the obesity and heart disease and diabetes epidemics, those guidelines have mostly made matters worse. We then got similarly terrible advice from the American Heart Association, American Dietetic Association, American Diabetes Association, and others. That advice has typically included:

- Obsessively focusing on tracking and controlling calories (typically not helpful to people and incredibly difficult to do).

- Carefully monitoring portion sizes and meticulously document everything we eat (a huge drain on our available resources, with notoriously inaccurate results).

- Very little attention paid to the importance of eating whole, unprocessed foods (probably the simplest and single most important factor in nutritional density).

- Zero emphasis on the *quality* of our calories, including where our food came from and how it was grown or raised.

- A lot of emphasis on avoiding fats in general, and saturated fats in particular, even though there's little decent science to support this counsel.[17] (Most of the science typically cited shows correlation vs. causation, or otherwise fails to separate nutrient-poor, processed food diets from whole-food diets that happen to be rich in whole-food fats.)

- Wrongheaded descriptions of saturated fats and red meat "clogging your arteries" (ignoring science that suggests arterial plaques are actually caused by inflammation and that both inflammation and elevated cholesterol are much more likely to be driven by diets high in refined carbohydrates, industrial oils, and other ultra-processed foods).

- Dire warnings about avoiding dietary cholesterol (which the USDA has now finally acknowledged is "not a nutrient of concern").

- Limited or delayed advice on avoiding trans fats, long after the science was clear on their dangers (this following two decades of public nutrition policies that actively promoted trans-fat-based margarines and spreads).[18]

- Encouragement to choose low-fat dairy products and "lean meats" over whole-fat options (again, with inadequate science to support this counsel).

- Aggressive promotion of polyunsaturated vegetable oils (known to drive inflammation and worsen our already dangerously imbalanced ratio of omega-6 and omega-3 fatty acids).

- Very little discussion of the role that phytonutrients (compounds found in plants) play in reducing inflammation, supporting immunity, and aiding in tissue repair, or the many intersecting roles that brightly colored, non-starchy vegetables play in supporting human health.

- Endless and aggressive promotion of whole grains, leading people to eat lots of breads and cereals made from flours, starches, and sugars—all of which quickly turn to sugar in the body, driving up insulin secretion and predisposing people to type 2 diabetes while crowding out much more nutritious, lower-glycemic load, non-starchy vegetables.

- Very little clarity on just how pervasive refined sugars and flours are in most processed foods (including many "whole-grain" products marketed as "healthy") and how responsible they are for unwanted weight gain and chronic inflammation.

- No discussion of the rising incidence of food intolerances to common substances like gluten, dairy, corn, soy, and eggs, or the role those intolerances can have in triggering or exacerbating common chronic diseases and conditions.

- No discussion of the problematic impact that food additives, including preservatives, emulsifiers, binders, artificial colors and flavors, can have on gut health.

I could go on. If you want the full litany of ways the USDA nutrition guidelines have run afoul of current science and ignored common sense, read Debra Minger's excellent (and disturbing) book, *Death by Food Pyramid*. Read Nina Teicholz's meticulously researched *Big Fat Surprise*. Or, for a quick snapshot of just how awful the advice being advanced by the powers-that-be really is, take a look at the *Diabetes Prevention Protocol Participant Handbook*.[19]

The product of vast sums of taxpayer money spent on the National Diabetes Prevention Program (National DPP), this initiative program has been rolled out to millions of people since it was created in 1996 and is today still promoted through hospitals, community health programs, and YMCAs.

In a section of the handbook labeled "Be a Fat and Calorie Detective," it offers all sorts of maddeningly counter-productive counsel like this:

To help you lose weight, we will begin building healthy eating habits. Here are some facts about fat and calories to get you started:

- Healthy eating means eating less fat and fewer calories.

- Eating too much fat is what makes us fat.

- By eating less, you can lose weight.

- Fat has the most calories of all the foods we eat. Fat contains more than twice the calories as the same amount of sugar, starch, or protein.

- Even small amounts of high-fat foods are high in calories.

Not true!

The text of this section goes on to tout the merits of eating three cups of air-popped popcorn rather than a quarter cup of peanuts (entirely on the basis of dietary fats and calories), and to generally blame type 2 diabetes on the overeating of fats rather than the insulin-disrupting, inflammatory effects of sugars, flours, and other refined carbohydrates. Throughout the handbook, the dietary advice is geared toward getting people to eat more whole grain breads and cereals. Meanwhile, much of the instruction sounds like it is coming from an imperious and condescending grade-school teacher:

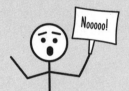

```
Write down everything you eat and drink.
It's the most important part of changing your behavior.
Spelling is not important. What is important is to:

• Be honest. Write down what you really eat.

• Be accurate. Measure portions,
  and read labels.

• Be complete. Include every little
  scrap you eat.
```

Blech. And again, it's not just *one* big, powerful organization doling out this sort of misguided advice. For decades, Americans have been getting similar counsel from the majority of large-scale health organizations, including the American Dietetic Association, American Heart Association, and the Centers for Disease Control. That advice has then been echoed, endlessly, by our society's most powerful and respected media outlets. It's been poured into textbooks, spooled out into public service announcements. It has, in effect, become "common knowledge."

By the way, this pattern of promoting ill-founded directives—typically requiring rigid self-control, delivering lackluster results, and leading to a cumulative undermining of health-motivated change—is by no means limited to the realm of diet and nutrition. It applies equally to how we've been told to exercise.

"Weight management," the CDC insists, "is all about balancing the number of calories you take in with the number your body uses or burns off." This oversimplified, mechanistic emphasis on caloric restriction and calorie-burning dominates most conventional health-improvement counsel. It ignores the fact that the *quality* and *kind* of calories you take in have everything to do with how many calories your body will burn as energy, and how many it will store as fat. It also ignores the fact that some calories inflame and fatigue your body, while others nourish and enliven it.

Similarly, in the weight-loss counsel from most conventional and "authoritative" sources, we rarely see any mention (much less any explanation) of the essential role that regular movement plays not just in calorie burning, but in virtually *every facet* of our body-mind well-being, including our energy, mood, circulation, metabolism, nervous system, detoxification, hormonal regulation, microbiome, immunity, and the expression of our DNA. Instead, all about "calories in, calories out." And that ham-handed explanation doesn't begin to do the complexity of the human body-mind systems justice.

The Hoodwinking of Health Seekers

You know what happens when millions of people are convinced to follow ineffective, counterproductive, and demoralizing approaches to health improvement? Exactly what's been happening the past few decades: Skyrocketing rates of obesity. Escalating levels of chronic inflammation and imbalance. Widespread human misery.

And what happens when we seek help for all these conditions of inflammation and imbalance within the conventional health-care system? We are given one or more official-sounding names for our particular collection of symptoms, and then encouraged to treat the symptoms (typically with drugs or medical procedures) rather than investigating and addressing the root causes of our distress.

This is the dynamic Jeffrey Bland, PhD, refers to in his excellent book, *The Disease Delusion,* as "the tyranny of the diagnosis." And the net result of this approach is not just that we spend three quarters of all our health-care dollars on ineffectively "managing" chronic diseases; it's that a huge percentage of our population is being oppressed by the physical, emotional, social, and financial burdens of complying with "health-care" advice that is in no way improving—*and may very well be worsening*—their health.

The longer we look to the Unhealthy Default Reality for solutions, the more disempowered, desperate, and deluded we become. To better understand how this works, let's consider two important psychological phenomena—ego depletion and learned helplessness—and how they work together to keep us stuck.

Ego Depletion

Have you ever noticed that your willpower tends to wane as the day wears on or that you're more inclined to gobble unhealthy snacks (or skip your evening workout or have an extra drink) on stressful days? That's ego depletion at work. The term *ego depletion* describes a fascinating body-mind dynamic by which what we think of as our willpower gets progressively depleted as the result of performing demanding tasks or enduring any sort of mental or emotional stress.[20]

It's been widely observed, both by social scientists and regular human beings standing in front of open refrigerators, that our mechanisms for self-discipline fluctuate moment to moment, day to day. Ego depletion explains why. It seems that each of us has a limited pool of self-regulatory mojo to pull from, and that mojo is depleted by all sorts of demands, trials, and tribulations. This includes the trials and tribulations that most of us face as we're navigating the Unhealthy Default Reality, day in and day out, from morning to night.

When studying ego depletion in formal experiments, psychologists have found that exposing test subjects to a mentally demanding task (like a math challenge or complex sorting exercise) before exposing them to a tempting food they are told to resist (like freshly baked chocolate chip cookies) reliably torpedoes their self-control.[21] It also works the other way around. When we are forced to exert a lot of self-control (whether in resisting cookies, trying to block out distractions, or striving to conceal our emotions), we tend to perform less well on virtually any subsequent test requiring significant draws on our mental, emotional, or physical resources.

Ego depletion isn't "just in your head." It has a clear biological basis, affecting and being affected by systems throughout your body, including blood sugar, heart-rate variability, immunity, and more. Basically, anything that demands attention, energy, and self-regulatory effort depletes your ability to apply those assets to other things—at least until you've had a chance to recover. It turns out that the kind of mental (brain) work required for intensive self-regulation consumes a great deal of glucose. That means it depletes blood sugar. And we know that having low blood sugar can have a huge impact on our mood and thinking, as well as our ability to exert willpower around what we eat. Ego depletion is just part of the reason (there are many others) why we are more inclined to eat poorly under stress, and also why following highly restrictive diets (even those that don't leave us physically hungry or nutrient deprived) tends to mess with our mind and our mood.

The High Costs of Restraint

There are a number of fascinating studies demonstrating that "restrained eaters" (those who carefully select their food in order to manage their weight or health) suffer from reduced cognitive capacity. You can see the most seminal of these studies referenced in a 2013 *Health Communication* journal article titled, "See the Seal? Understanding Restrained Eaters' Responses to Nutritional Messages on Food Packaging."[22] And it is an article worth reading, because once you've seen how restrained eating impedes cognition, you begin to understand what a Catch-22 health seeking has become.

Compared to more freewheeling eaters, this article explains, restrained eaters tend to exhibit "lower levels of sustained attention, recall, and working memory" and are "more likely to engage in rapid or heuristic rather than more detailed and systematic processing of packaging information including seals and claims." Worn down by their self-restraint efforts, such eaters appear more inclined to "engage in information search truncation." This means that even though they intend to make thoughtful eating decisions, they are more likely to wind up limiting their attention to front-of-label claims (e.g., "sugar-free," "gluten-free," "low calorie") or to rely on seals of approval for guidance, rather than review the ingredients and nutrition panel for more substantive information. This, the study authors explain, "may lead restrained eaters to reach different healthfulness judgments and purchase-intention outcomes from unrestrained eaters."

What a horrible irony. The harder you work at making tightly regulated, strictly healthy selections, the more cognitively depleted you become, and the more vulnerable to choosing a health-hyped product that doesn't actually meet your intended standards. Note that this is not just true of food choices. Typically, the more brain power and willpower we are using to regulate any part of our decision making in one area, the less capable we will be of making complex, carefully reasoned, or self-regulated decisions in other areas.

You probably know this willpower-depletion dynamic from experience. And, knowing what you now know about the Unhealthy Default Reality, you can probably see why this dynamic poses an intractable problem for most of us. Just to make it super clear, though, I'm going to break it down, step-by-nasty-step:

- The UDR exposes us to an endless series of challenging, draining, and stressful experiences, including many inherent to our unprecedented state of evolutionary mismatch.

- The UDR also exposes us to an endless series of designed-to-be-addictive modern temptations, overwhelming consumer options, and Unhealthy Default Choices.

- The UDR constantly broadcasts messages telling us that we're not good enough, that we don't look right, aren't choosing right, and aren't living up to expectations (more stress).

- The UDR then suggests that we must eat healthy and exercise in order to counter our unhealthy circumstances and that we need to buy a bunch of things and do a bunch of things to embrace a "healthy lifestyle" (more demands, more consumer choices, more stress).

- A lot of those healthy-lifestyle prescriptions don't work, don't work in the context of our UDR-dictated lives, can't be done on the dwindling supply of self-regulatory resources we have left—or they just plain backfire (creating an additional series of challenging, draining, and stressful experiences).

- We're told (explicitly or implicitly) that we just need to have more willpower *or* we're told we have a disease (or more than one disease) and that we must rely on conventional medicine for solutions.

- Those conventional medical solutions (drugs and procedures) often result in additional drains on our physical, mental, emotional, and financial resources (and more stress).

Even though millions of other people are suffering the same fate, it is rarely acknowledged by any of the powers that be (government, mainstream media, experts) that the way we are living is entirely out of sync with our DNA—the DNA that runs every single one of our cells, including the ones in our brains.

Basically, as noted in chapter 2, the UDR obstructs our view of our historical past, distorts our view of our current reality, then exposes us to stresses for which we are in no way prepared, then drains every ounce of willpower we have by every means at its disposal, then demands that we tightly regulate our behavior and exert extraordinary levels of self-control, then gives us lousy advice about how we should be using what little self-control we have left, then reminds us a thousand times a day that we are failing, then offers us an incredible array of anesthetizing and depleting (and inflammatory) distractions, then heaps on more challenges, more demands, and more temptations, and then demands to know why the #%@$ we aren't keeping pace.

Dah! It's no wonder we're all struggling!

You probably know from watching the news (which I don't recommend, by the way) and hearing about an endless stream of high-profile overdoses, arrests, hospitalizations, and suicides that even celebrities and rich people are struggling. So, it's really important to understand: *This is not your problem with self-control and willpower. This is our shared, endemic problem with chronic depletion and distraction.*

It's time for us to openly acknowledge, to ourselves and others, that we have been asking the near impossible of ourselves and others. It's time to acknowledge, as Albert Einstein so wisely did, that we cannot solve our problems using the same level of thinking that created them. When we allow the UDR to convince us that our commonly experienced health and self-breakage problems are entirely the result of our personal shortcomings, and when we accept the crappy, counterproductive solutions the UDR has to offer, it sets us up for forever trying and failing. And that leads to a phenomenon known as *learned helplessness.*

Learned Helplessness

The studies on learned helplessness are nasty even to read about. Ironically, the earliest and most seminal of these studies were conducted by Martin Seligman, PhD, a researcher widely considered to be one of the pioneers of positive psychology. I say "ironically" because while positive psychology is, at least in principle, the study of mental wellness (as opposed to the study of illness and dysfunction, which are the domain of conventional psychology), in their quest for answers, positive psychologists have resorted to some pretty sadistic and insanity-inducing research experiments.

Seligman's studies into learned helplessness, for example, involved restraining individual dogs in harnesses and then subjecting them to painful electric shocks. Some of the dogs in these studies were given an opportunity to stop the shocks by pushing a panel with their noses. Others had no means of controlling the shocks, and thus no choice but to endure them. Once the dogs were conditioned in this way, the researchers placed them inside restricted environments called shuttle boxes. These boxes had two sides separated by an adjustable wall. The researchers could control which side (or sides) of the enclosure would deliver electric shocks, and could also raise or lower the height of the wall in order to control the animal's options for shock avoidance.

I'll simplify the description of these experiments because (1) they're horrible (the shocks were painful enough, according to Seligman, to cause the dogs to yelp, whimper, and spontaneously soil themselves); and (2) all the details and variables of the studies would take too long to explain. Basically, though, the studies involved seeing how dogs with different types of preconditioning would respond to a variety of shock and shock-avoidance scenarios.

The outcomes were disturbing. The dogs that had been conditioned to believe they could stop the shocks were able to learn quite rapidly in this new scenario that by hopping over a low wall when prompted, they could avoid additional negative stimulus (shocks). The dogs conditioned toward helplessness, however, behaved very differently. After a brief period of darting around within the electrified shuttle box, these dogs would just give up, lie down, and accept their miserable fate.

To be clear, at this point, these poor creatures had the exact same opportunities as their more hopeful peers to scramble over a low wall and escape the source of their suffering, but as a result of their preconditioning, they behaved as though they did not. Having learned from previous experiences that there was no point in trying to avoid the shocks, these dogs would simply lie there and submit to them, flinching and whimpering, rather than making any effort at escape.

A lot of animal studies have been done on learned helplessness, and they have all gone about the same way. I won't subject you to more descriptions of them, because they make me sad and upset. But I will share one interesting and important point with you. It turns out that decades of studies on learned helplessness, while diverse in their methods and scenarios, tend to produce surprisingly consistent conclusions—not just in dogs and rats, but also in people:

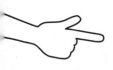

Once an individual has succumbed to a state of learned helplessness, that state tends to stubbornly persist.

Animal researchers have found, in fact, that there is only one reliable way to convince a creature convinced of its helplessness to reassert agency over its well-being, and that is to force its body through self-rescuing actions. In Seligman's studies, for example, when researchers attempted to un-train the dogs they had just brainwashed into a state of learned helplessness, they only managed to do so by putting leashes around the dogs' necks and repeatedly dragging them to the shock-free sides of their shuttle boxes.

Over time, thank goodness, the dogs got the message, and researchers found they could dial back their force, shifting from forcibly dragging the animals to more gently tugging or nudging them to move. Finally, with repeated training and practice, these animals were reacquainted with the strategic art of pain avoidance. But this was not some quickly grasped "aha" moment on the part of the dogs. On the contrary, in order to shake off the helplessness imposed upon them, they had to have their body-minds aggressively retrained in the motions required for autonomous escape.

Hmm. These are important lessons for those of us living in the proverbial cages of the UDR. First, because most of us have had our own share of the UDR's lessons in learned helplessness (unrelenting problems, ineffective solutions), and second, because even if we *could* somehow manage to extract all the right how-to-escape info from the UDR (exactly what to eat and exactly how to move, manage stress, and get enough sleep), it seems clear that just being *told* what to do and how to do it is probably not going to be enough. We may, at least initially, need to have our body-minds moved into self-rescuing action.

This is the idea behind the Healthy Deviant Adventure program in part 4. While this program will not drag you by the neck, it will gently guide your body-mind through the motions of escape, deftly retraining it in the autonomous actions required to escape the cage-like constraints of the UDR.

Okay, just a couple more points. First, I want to reassure you that it is unlikely you are currently in a full state of learned helplessness (because if you were, you would probably not be reading this book). Then again, compulsively consuming self-help literature *can be* a symptom of UDR entrapment, and also one of its slipperiest mechanisms for keeping us stuck. Diving in and out of lots of different plans and protocols (particularly when none of them are working for you) can be yet another drain on your self-regulatory reserves. And the instant-solution-seeking, "fix-me" mentality our society loves to promote is one of those same-level-thinking constructs that simply cannot solve the problems it produced.

So, before we go further, I want to offer you a little more insight on why simply willing or forcing yourself through the motions of any program, even mine, is unlikely to produce great results. The real magic happens when you decide to do some small thing differently and then *start paying attention to what happens next.*

Working Around Willpower

There is a massive body of scientific research suggesting that what we think of as willpower is one of the single biggest predictive traits (second, perhaps, only to intelligence) in determining life success. I'm going to take some issue with those findings shortly, but first, allow me to give that notion its due.

It's not difficult to see how willpower-as-success-determinant would make sense from an evolutionary perspective. In our hunter-gatherer days, having the self-control to stay perfectly still while lying low in itchy grass would increase your ability to take down your prey. Having the self-control to not eat the entire day's haul of foraged berries while walking back to camp would work both to your social advantage and to the advantage of your tribe's survival (which would be closely tied to your own). Given this, it's not hard to imagine that individuals with higher levels of self-regulatory capacity stood a far better chance of surviving, thriving, mating, and successfully passing on their genes (which, from an evolutionary standpoint, is the only success that matters).

It's also clear that our forebears had some significant willpower advantages over us modern-day humans. First, they had endless opportunity to continuously build and maintain their self-regulatory mojo. Every day brought opportunities to do difficult but important, socially supported tasks that required great focus and persistence, from traveling long distances on foot and tolerating broad extremes of temperature to skinning animals with stone tools and starting fires by hand. Meanwhile, unlike us, our ancestors were *not* exposed to the sorts of modern-day stresses, temptations, decisions, and sensory overloads (fast-food drive-thrus, Cinnabon stands, video games, advertising, the internet, shopping malls)[23] in which we find ourselves continuously enmeshed.

You can see how all of this would have made it a whole lot easier for our ancestors to conserve, practice, and wisely allocate their willpower reserves for the times when it really mattered. In our not-so-distant hunter-gatherer past, thanks to 2.5 million years of adaptation, it seems likely that our supplies of willpower were nicely adapted to the full scope of willpower-demanding situations we faced on a daily basis. Now, however, in the face of the UDR, our DNA-conferred supplies of willpower have become hopelessly inadequate.

In much the same way that our ancestrally programmed, calorie-thrifty metabolisms were ideal for surviving famines but left us ill-prepared to deal with today's sugar-drenched, calorie-unlimited environments, our evolutionarily mismatched willpower-deployment mechanisms (developed over the same 2.5-million-year time frame) have left us equally ill-prepared for our unprecedented modern-day straits.

This brings me to one of the most fundamental principles of Healthy Deviance:

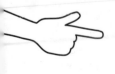

In the context of the Unhealthy Default Reality, relying on willpower is an unwise strategy.

Leaning too hard on willpower sets us up for that vicious cycle in which we try to resist unrelenting streams of temptation and overstimulation, get depleted from our efforts, fail, feel stressed and ashamed about our failure (more ego depletion), commence to try harder, and so on. After a number of rounds of that, we sink into a state of learned helplessness. Like Seligman's misery-conditioned dogs, we eventually become inured to our own suffering, and seeing no means of escape, we start to feel resigned to our fate. Eventually, we may simply stop trying.

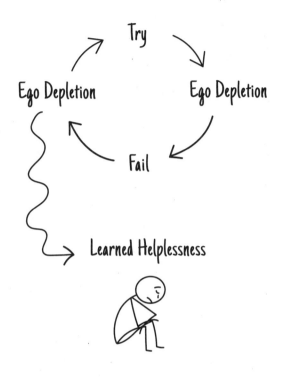

This is precisely why ego depletion is the UDR's favorite weapon. The more complex decisions and temptations it can throw at us, and the more stress it can expose us to, the lousier and less certain it can make us feel about our choices, and the better chance it has of immobilizing us in a state of vulnerability.

Remember, too, that ego depletion grinds down our mental capacity. The preeminent willpower researcher Roy Baumeister, PhD, explains it this way: "As you make a bunch of decisions, you gradually deplete the energy you have available." As a result, he notes, your subsequent decisions become "more passive," and you become more inclined to "go with the default option."

In the Unhealthy Default Reality, we know what the passive, default option will be: unhealthy and depleting—an express-lane on-ramp to a whole series of other unhealthy default choices. So I want to emphasize this again. *In the Unhealthy Default Reality, asking people to manage health-determining decisions via willpower is a setup for failure.*

And yet, insanely, that is precisely what we do. It's what we ask of ourselves and our children. It's what we expect of others. Despite mountains of research showing this plainly does not work, after decades of ineffective efforts and billions of dollars spent trying to get people to avoid, by sheer willpower, the unhealthy behaviors our society made easy in the first place, we seem determined to continue on that course.

We have, I think, reached the "bread and circus" phase of our society's development in this realm. The bulk of popular attention is focused squarely on the superficial trappings and signifiers of health and fitness ("Your best body ever!" "Clear skin NOW!") even as the difficulty of providing for our most essential needs becomes ever more pronounced. While our health-care system is consumed with "managing" chronic diseases, our entire culture and consumer economy is wired up to aggressively fuel them.

Societally, our response to widespread chronic illness and misery amounts not just to rearranging the deck chairs on the Titanic but also to having them sent out to be reupholstered and paying a rush charge to get them back before the ship sinks. Clearly, that's no good. So, what's a better strategy?

First, if we want to stand any chance of summoning willpower adequate to the environments we find ourselves in now, we have to *choose our willpower expenditures with great care and discernment,* assiduously fending off leaks and poor uses.

Second, we have to do things that help us *actively build our genetically predetermined stores of willpower and develop our willpower-deployment mechanisms* to meet our current demands.

This means:

- Structuring your life in such a way that you preemptively manage your stores of energy and attention, and anticipating and noticing the many ways in which the UDR will always be actively sapping them.

- Avoiding any and all unnecessary exposure to the stream of temptations and distractions the UDR cranks out (like media, retail environments, and other stimuli-saturated surroundings).

- Using your willpower strategically to do smart, high-octane things proven to help you build your willpower muscles and maintain your autonomy, even in the face of the UDR's persistent attempts to rob you of it (see parts 3 and 4 for practical guidance on this).

- Preemptively minimizing your background and peripheral requirements for willpower, while proactively building "back-up stores" that you can direct in whatever ways and moments you choose.

Needless to say, doing all of these things does, in itself, require a certain amount of willpower and cognitive capacity. But these are the *right* places to invest whatever willpower and cognitive capacity you have. First, because research suggests that making self-directed, values-driven, intrinsically motivated choices like these doesn't deplete you in the same way that resisting chocolate chip cookies can (look up "self-determination therapy" for more on that). And second, because the alternative—living in a way that requires you to take your chances with the vagaries of the UDR almost guarantees you won't have enough willpower to bring to bear when you really need it.

Mojo Generation and Depletion

This brings us to an interesting question. Where does this thing we call *willpower* actually come from? What is it, really? How can we best hope to harness it and dispense it wisely?

Both from my own experience and from the troves of research I have read on the topic over my two decades as a health journalist, I've come to the conclusion that "willpower" is really just an expression of our available energy, vitality, clarity, confidence, and resilience. Basically, it's a reflection of our available mojo at a given time.

By *mojo,* I mean our sense of personal energy, power, and autonomy—our capacity to make self-determining decisions that serve our highest goals and values. So, what dictates our available level of mojo? Three main categories of things, all of which are tightly interrelated:

1. **Our central physiological status:** Blood sugar. Organ reserves. Energy stores. Microbiome balance.[24] Immunity.[25] Basic physical vitality.

2. **Our current neurological wiring and firing:** The density, arrangement, and health of our brain circuitry (neurons, dendrites, synaptic networks), the activation levels of various locations in our brain, and the way that circuitry is inclined to fire (reactively and instinctively versus via executive function).

3. **Our mental, emotional, social, and spiritual state:** Our attitudes, ideas, conditioning, priorities, values, belief systems, and sense of self-regard, as well as the place these things currently hold in our conscious awareness.

Okay, so what dictates the rate at which our mojo is depleted? Two things:

1. **Exposure to distracting, demanding, painful, stressful, disempowering, willpower-draining situations:** The more of them we're dealing with, the less mojo we have to deal with anything else.

2. **Our attitude, preparedness, and competence in recognizing and dealing with those situations:** The more quickly we can recognize that a particular circumstance is messing with us, and the more advanced our skills and confidence in problem-solving, the less we'll allow our mojo to be drained before taking evasive or corrective action.

The problem, of course, is that the average person living in the Unhealthy Default Reality has to spend hours on end resisting temptations and striving to self-regulate under stressful conditions while *also* battling a lot of distractions from background stimulus.

This means your mojo is, by default, depleted all day long, day in and day out, year after year.

As a result of getting subpar nutrition, being exposed to all sorts of toxins, and getting inadequate or overly stressful exercise, the average person living in the Unhealthy Default Reality is also *physically* depleted, inflamed, hormonally disrupted, and biochemically imbalanced virtually all of the time. So unless you take aggressive evasive actions in the moments when you still have your physical reserves and mental synapses on board, and unless you are also constantly replenishing those reserves and safeguarding those synapses, there's only one way this can play out: You are going to be one hurting, mojo-depleted unit, chronically vulnerable to temptations and poor decisions of all kinds.

Gah! Okay, I think that covers the problems. Let's move onto the solutions.

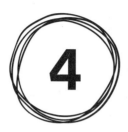

The Renegade Solution

You never change things by fighting the existing reality.
To change something, build a new model
that makes the existing model obsolete.

—R. BUCKMINSTER FULLER

Ready to slip the trap that's been laid for you and step into a better, more radiant, and more resilient way of living? The rest of this book shows you how to craft your own escape route from the Unhealthy Default Reality (UDR) *and* have a really good time doing it.

By now, I'm hoping you are getting a sense of why conventional diet-and-exercise and other "willpower" interventions don't work very well, at least not for very long or for very many. Most of us are simply starting from a too-depleted, too-distracted, too-compromised position to summon the huge self-regulatory powers required to maintain those interventions. Even when we do have momentary success—following the requisite diet or doing the must-do workout or achieving the must-have look—the efforts required for that too often come out of dangerously low reserves, weakening us in other ways, and throwing us back into the red zone of our own emptiness.

As a rule, the more of ourselves we give over to the UDR, the stronger it gets and the weaker we get. Our well-meaning endeavors, our earnest applications of effort and attention, only serve to reinforce the machine. To break free of this cycle, you have to do two things:

- Remember that the problem is not you; it's the UDR.

- Embrace only solutions geared to that problem. By that I mean, cease trying to fix your perceived flaws and shortcomings, and instead begin adjusting how you relate to the UDR.

Okay, so what's a good way of relating to the UDR? Well, rather than seeing yourself as being victimized or oppressed by it (even if that seems evidently true), I suggest embracing the UDR as a worthy foe, one that's giving you an endless series of opportunities to become stronger, clearer, and more creative with time and experience (for more on that, see day 3 of the Healthy Deviant Adventure program, "Find Things Right"). Seen through a Healthy Deviant's eyes, every encounter with the UDR is an opportunity to:

- Increase your awareness, focus, clarity of thought.

- Reduce your vulnerability, reactivity, and impulsivity.

- Build your capacity, knowledge, and skill.

- Expand your sense of potential and purpose.

In short, every day is an invitation to turn the vicious cycle of the Unhealthy Default Reality on its head and to begin establishing the virtuous cycle of Healthy Deviance in its place. The virtuous cycle of Healthy Deviance looks like this.

Virtuous Cycle of Healthy Deviance

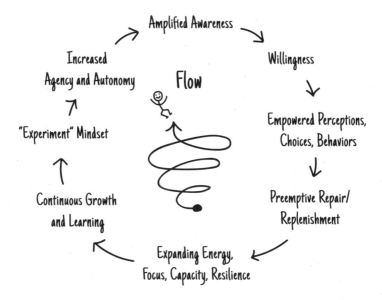

Amplified Awareness

Increased Agency and Autonomy

Flow

Willingness

"Experiment" Mindset

Empowered Perceptions, Choices, Behaviors

Continuous Growth and Learning

Preemptive Repair/ Replenishment

Expanding Energy, Focus, Capacity, Resilience

You'll note that whereas the vicious cycle of the UDR calls on you to exert an endless amount of willpower, the virtuous cycle of Healthy Deviance calls upon you to:

- Raise your level of awareness.

- Cultivate the willingness to preemptively, continuously build and defend your stores of energy, clarity, vitality.

- Develop your ability to monitor and allocate the resources you have on tap at any given time.

- Anticipate, based on past experience, when your self-regulatory resources will be most needed and/or in short supply.

- Design your life and develop skill sets in ways that minimize your requirements for "willpower" and help avoid unnecessary drains on your energy reserves.

The goal here is to amass enough surplus energy and vitality (mojo) that you can navigate safely within the UDR. I'm going to suggest you begin by practicing some super-simple Renegade Rituals (see part 3 for descriptions and directions). As you perform these rituals, you're going to start noticing what it feels like to pull yourself out of the danger zone of depletion and into a better-fueled state of body-mind resilience.

First, you'll gauge and honestly acknowledge where you currently are on your own energy and vitality meter, even if that's someplace you'd prefer not to be, like this ...

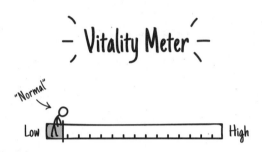

Next, you'll begin taking some simple steps (like the Renegade Rituals and other suggested exercises in this book) to extract yourself.

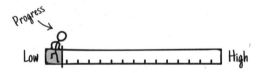

Then, you'll begin envisioning where you are headed next, even if that is simply a state of incremental progress and learning.

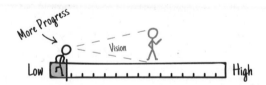

Then, as you build energy and confidence, you'll begin to envision yourself in an even better place.

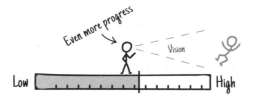

And, eventually, you'll find yourself at a place that previously would have been hard for you to imagine.

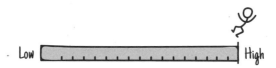

At some point, when you get healthy and happy enough, you'll realize your entire scale of expectation and hope has expanded. You'll discover you've got capacity and potential you didn't even realize was available to you.

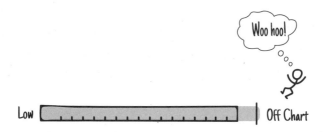

I'll go into more detail about all of this in part 3. And then, in part 4, over the course of the Healthy Deviant Adventure program, you'll have a chance to try it all out on yourself, if you choose. The Daily Deviance Journal Pages and Healthy Deviant Adventure Tracker will give you an easy way to keep track of how your Vitality Meter is reading on any given day and to begin noticing the patterns in its fluctuations.

For now, though, let's focus on the more urgent task at hand, which is blowing up the experiment in which you've been trapped so you can begin the self-extraction process in earnest.

Blowing Up the Experiment

You know that ego depletion experiment with the chocolate chip cookies I told you about back in chapter 3? The researchers made a point of not telling the people in the experiment that resisting them was a test of their willpower or even a central component of the research being conducted. Instead, they lied to them, giving them some false reason not to eat the cookies (saying they were going to be used for a different experiment, for example).

Why the deception? Because the researchers knew full well that having the subjects *understand* the true purpose and framework of the experiment would skew the results. When people are told that their willpower is being evaluated, they will generally focus all their attention on the willpower-related task at hand (even if that means they will have less to expend elsewhere later). In other words, if you are aware of the circumstances, you can decide what matters enough to deserve your willpower, and then redirect it accordingly.

The problem is, nobody is going to remind you on a daily basis that you are living in the midst of a giant experiment that is rigged to suck you dry of all your resources. Nobody is going to tell you that you are being tested to see how well you can conserve those resources for your own sanity and well-being. So I am telling you now:

You are the subject of an experiment.

Seriously. You are. First, as noted, you are the first generation in human history to have lived in circumstances anything like the ones you are living in now. You are that ape in the arcade (discussed in chapter 3). Second, your ability to monitor and strategically allocate your mental, emotional, and physical resources under these unprecedented circumstances is being tested and challenged—actively—by industries and institutions that have a major stake in getting you to do and buy certain things.

Your consumer behavior, your media preferences, every subtle nuance of your desires and priorities is constantly being surveyed, monitored, split-tested, and manipulated by people who stand to make millions from getting you to want more, need more, crave more, click more, worry more, and spend more. Every shift of your attitudes and appetites is constantly being observed by institutions that have a vested stake in making you feel progressively less certain that anything about you and your life is as it should be.

As the result of being experimented on in this way, you may very well be feeling anxious, depressed, fatigued, depleted and like you have zero energy or vitality to spare. Or, at least, not as much as you would like. To change that, you have to pull your energy back from the experimenters. You must devise experiments of your own to see how successfully you can ward off the vitality-sapping forces of the UDR and reclaim you own agency and autonomy for your own purposes.

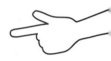

You must wriggle your way out of the experimental trap you are in.

I can tell you this, and I will, many times throughout this book. But ultimately, you need to remind yourself. Daily. Proactively. Repeatedly. "You are being experimented on." Until it becomes background knowledge. Until it becomes your habitual way of doing business with the UDR. Until the UDR loses its grip on you. At that point, you'll have blown up the experiment you've been subjected to and, instead, be living in an experiment of your own design—an experiment in Healthy Deviance, which is a much nicer place to be.

Where Affirmations and Visualizations Meet Action

Within the field of popular psychology, there's an ongoing argument about the value of wishful thinking versus willful action. One school argues (in the style of Deepak Chopra, MD, and Rhonda Byrne's *The Secret*) that with enough positive affirmations and visualizations, change will happen, with little effort, through some invisible force. Another school argues (in the style of psychology researcher Roy Baumeister, PhD) that willpower is king and that "just doing" a thing is the only way to get it done.

In my mind, these two schools aren't really opposed: First, thinking positive thoughts and visualizing desired states *is* doing a thing. And it's a *super important* thing, because it helps rewire the neurocircuitry in our brains in ways that predispose us to taking positive action. It helps build our stores of available energy, and it helps ward off learned helplessness. Doing outward, active, physical things helps too, because action-oriented steps build our willpower muscles in a host of different ways. For example, consider the following:

- Taking even minuscule, low-effort steps in the direction of our goals helps build self-efficacy.

- Setting up our environments in ways that minimize friction, distraction, and temptation helps break down resistance and predisposes us toward desired actions and attitudes.

- Leveraging low-effort foundational habits builds confidence and self-regard, creating physical and mental on-ramps toward the successful pursuit of tougher changes.

- Making positive changes in our physical nourishment and activity can shift our microbiome, immunity, blood sugar levels, cell function, and other biochemical factors that play a huge role in our mood, focus, and ability to self-regulate.

So it's really not a matter of either/or. It's a matter of both/and (in whatever combinations you feel most willing to embrace now).

A number of studies—including many from Yale University, the University of California at Los Angeles, and the Center for Healthy Minds at the University of Wisconsin, Madison—have shown that meditation and positive visualizations can help us lay down new neural networks, changing the infrastructure of our brains and thereby helping shift our sense of agency and identity. Some research has even shown that meditation can influence the expression of our DNA.[26] Conducting real-life experiments, meanwhile, helps us challenge our limiting beliefs and engrained patterns in visceral ways that simply imagining or visualizing those things cannot. Taking action provides confirming evidence of desired-state affirmations.

It's one thing to regularly repeat a daily affirmation like "I'm healthy and whole." It's another to say, with clarity and confidence, "I am a person who walks in the morning," and to know this is true—even if that walk starts out as just the twelve steps to the mailbox and back.

From Death Grip to Refillable Cup

Many of the Healthy Deviant solutions I am proposing have to do with shifting your focus from willpower to willingness, and shifting your priorities from fixing your flaws to building up your mojo. I realize all of this can sound rather vague and conceptual, so to get a more practical, kinetic sense of what I'm suggesting you do, try this two-part exercise I call "Shifting Your Grip."

"SHIFTING YOUR GRIP" EXERCISE: PART 1

Hold your arm out straight in front of you and make a fist. Clench it hard, imagining that in your fist, you hold your willpower. This is the willpower required to do all the things you have to do in order to be healthy and successful—eat right, exercise, get enough sleep, be organized, resist temptation—so you must do everything you can to keep that willpower locked within your closed hand.

Imagine it is like a handful of sand. If you loosen your grip, it will seep out. You'll have failed, lost, proven yourself inadequate. Game over.

Try walking around with your extended hand clenched like that and notice how much it demands from your entire body. Feel the tension that builds in your arm, and how it starts to radiate through the rest of your body. Is your jaw tight? Your shoulder? Your neck? Is your other hand tensing or clenching automatically? How about your toes? Is your head jutting forward? Are you holding your breath?

Once you have a clear sense of how much exertion and mental focus it demands from your whole body-mind to keep your fist so tight, I want you to take a moment to imagine how hard it would be to do anything else while in this state. That is what relying on willpower feels like. This is what it feels like to be forever fighting and correcting your "flaws."

Not fun. Blech.

"SHIFTING YOUR GRIP" EXERCISE: PART 2

Okay, now, drop your arm to your side, relax your clenched fist, relax your willpower muscles, and let the imaginary sand fall from your hand onto the floor. Just let it go. You don't need it. Wiggle your fingers. Close your eyes. Shake out your body. Take a breath, and just release all the tension you've built up.

Whew! That's better, right?

Now, keeping your elbow at your side, bring your hand back up in front of you so the pinky side of your hand is just gently grazing your belly button. Hold your hand, palm up, in a relaxed, gently cupped shape. Feel how much less tension and focus it requires to hold this position. Walk around a bit, and notice how much easier it is to use the other parts of your body while keeping your arm lightly engaged.

Next, imagine there's a little pool of water in your hand. Keep moving. Notice that even if your pool of water were to slosh out or evaporate as you move, with your hand open like this, it would be very easy to fill back up without ever changing your position. You could also refill it with whatever other substance you like, whatever serves you at a given time. Maybe sand. Maybe water. Maybe chocolate. Maybe wine.

This is what engaging willingness and building your mojo feels like.

Compared to squeezing that fistful of sand, this water-holding exercise still requires attention, but not so much exertion. It involves engagement, flexibility, freedom, and self-directed power. Moving through life this way requires more awareness, less effort. It presents a series of opportunities to notice and choose.

This is the difference between willpower and willingness, between flaw fixing and mojo building. And this, in essence, is the positional shift I'll be inviting you to experiment with from here on out.

From clenching to holding lightly.
From fighting loss to refilling often.
From exhausting yourself to enjoying yourself.
Amen.

From Learned Helplessness to Flow

Part of what makes willingness-based refilling easy is that it's an inherently gratifying state to be in. If the vicious cycle of the Unhealthy Default Reality both feeds on and produces learned helplessness, the virtuous cycle of Healthy Deviance both draws on and results in a state of flow.

Flow, a concept put forth by positive psychologist Mihaly Csikszentmihalyi, is a sought-after state of "intrinsic" motivation and "autotelic" reward, the kind that originates from within. Flow, in Csikszentmihalyi's words, is characterized by "being completely involved in an activity for its own sake."

Flow states are typically produced by activities that share the following characteristics:

- They challenge and stretch your available skills, but they are not so difficult or impossible that they become frustrating or incline you to give up.

- They require intense focus, high engagement, and close attention to the activity or task at hand.

- They feature clear goals or parameters of success and produce gratifying results you deem worthwhile.

- They give you the sense that you are making adequate progress against a known goal, that you are in control of the outcome.

- They cause you to feel absorbed, transported, and to lose any sense of self-consciousness or insecurity, as well as your sense of time.

- They feel inherently rewarding, deeply satisfying, sometimes even euphoric, resulting in a self-perpetuating desire to continue with the activity.

While in a flow state, Csikszentmihalyi explains, "The ego falls away. Time flies. Every action, movement, and thought follows inevitably from the previous one, like playing jazz. Your whole being is involved, and you're using your skills to the utmost."[27] Flow states can also have their downside (namely, that they can become addictive if done to excess or to the exclusion of other life priorities), but they are generally seen as producing both happy humans and good collateral results.

Is it possible to make Healthy Deviance—the collection of acts and attitudes required to be healthy in an unhealthy world—into an ongoing series of periodic flow states? I think so. In my experience, Healthy Deviance presents the opportunity for flow states galore, and for the Healthy Deviants I've witnessed doing their thing, flow certainly seems to be a common experience.

Let's consider the key components and competencies of Healthy Deviance in relationship to the requirements of Csikszentmihalyi's flow state:

Challenging, requires full application of your available skill (but is not frustrating or beyond reach) ...

Check. The first challenge of Healthy Deviance involves switching gears from willpower to willingness. From there, as you build and apply an increasing array of healthy living skills, you raise your game and take on bigger challenges. You define the game. You constantly adjust so you are playing at, but not beyond, the limit of your current skills. If you are feeling frustrated or helpless, you are either depleted or playing beyond your current level—or both. All you have to do is take a step back and reengage with the basics. Drink a glass of water. Eat a vegetable. Go stand outdoors for a minute. Take some deep breaths. Okay, you are back in the game, and *back in charge* of the game.

Involves focus, engagement, close attention ...

Check. Healthy Deviance calls for you to be fully present, actively directing your attention, closely monitoring your present condition, and aggressively defending yourself against distractions and incursions. The UDR never sleeps, never idles, never ceases trying to tap into your databanks and resource reserves. When you lose focus and fall prey to the UDR (which will typically be a zillion times a day), you can notice the telltale signs and either regather your attention, or recognize that you no longer have any, and then take a break to replenish your capacity. When you wind up drop-kicked or sucker-punched by the UDR, you can pay attention to how that happened.[28]

Features a clear goal or parameters of success, produces gratifying results ...

Check. You want to be a healthy person in an unhealthy world. Any step you take in that direction, anything you learn, any way you grow, any way you avoid falling into the gaping maw of the UDR (or even notice that you have fallen in) represents success. Every moment of progress, increased awareness, or healthy pleasure represents a gratifying result that is yours for the claiming.

Gives you the sense you are making progress against your goal ...

Check. To the extent you are making progress, you are winning. If you are not making progress, but noticing that and investigating the patterns behind your lack of progress, you are also winning. When you overshoot your current capacity, you get feedback. And when you notice and incorporate that feedback, you win again. In other words, you are in the process of winning all of the time.

Feels deeply satisfying, sometimes even euphoric, resulting in a self-perpetuating desire to continue with the activity ...

Check. Check. Check. The experience of pausing to notice your present condition, of choosing to respond thoughtfully and non-reactively to your body-mind's current needs, is an inherently creative and pleasurable practice. Each time you make a self-respecting, self-supporting choice, you experience a return of energy and enthusiasm, a surge of self-efficacy, an amplified sense of vitality, and the divine satisfaction knowing you've just outwitted the UDR. These intrinsic rewards perpetuate your desire to continue.

Okay, What Now?

You have a couple options at this point:

1. You can continue on and read part 2, "The Making of a Healthy Deviant" (in which I share my own Healthy Hero's Journey and help you find your place in yours).

2. You can skip directly to part 3, "The Way of the Healthy Deviant," and begin learning about the Nonconformist Competencies and Renegade Rituals of Healthy Deviance.

   If you skip to part 3, I hope you'll come back and read part 2 at some point, because a big part of it is your story, and you're the only one who can decide how it goes from here.

   Either way, before you do anything else, I invite you to complete the Weird Symptom Checklist on the next page.

Weird Symptom Checklist

The human body has a fascinating language for expressing its discontent, distress, depletion, and dis-ease. How many of the following signals is your body sending you?

As you review the list below, check the ones that sound familiar. Also note how long you've been experiencing them.

☐ Unwanted weight gain or loss
☐ Increasing fat stores around your abdomen, or development of a pot belly
☐ Rashes, including eczema and psoriasis plaques, or red, scaly patches behind ears
☐ Acne, cysts, rosacea, and inflamed skin
☐ Small sores, cysts, or pimples at base of neck, around jawline
☐ Puffy face, swollen hands, feet, and ankles
☐ Stuffy, drippy, or congested nasal passages
☐ Itchiness or tickly feeling inside ears and throat
☐ Hair thinning, loss, and dullness (head, body, eyelashes, and brows)
☐ Dandruff, athlete's foot, toenail fungus, or yeast infections

☐ Brittle, weak, flaking, ridged, pitted, spotted, or misshapen fingernails
☐ Bleeding or inflamed gums
☐ Coated, spotted, fissured, "bald," or scalloped tongue
☐ Dry, flaking skin (all over or just in patches) or raised, rough bumps
☐ Crepe-y skin, dull complexion, loss of skin sheen or "glow"
☐ Dark circles or semi-circles of puffiness under eyes
☐ Watery or red-rimmed eyes, or eyes with bloodshot, greyish, or yellowish whites
☐ Cracked and peeling lips
☐ Tongue bumps, mouth sores, cracking at corners of mouth
☐ Bad breath
☐ Night sweats
☐ Difficulty getting to sleep or sleeping through the night
☐ Difficulty waking up in the morning
☐ Fatigue, low endurance for physical activity
☐ Feeling "blah," "meh," or otherwise uninspired
☐ Depression, moodiness, irritation, or lack of patience
☐ Brain fog, difficulty focusing, or slowed thinking
☐ Racing heart, rapid pulse, or irregular heartbeat

- ☐ Facial tics or eye fluttering
- ☐ Frequent headaches (including migraines or cluster headaches)
- ☐ Chronic musculoskeletal pain, stiffness, or tension (back of head, neck, back, joint)
- ☐ Obsessive-compulsive behaviors (cuticle picking, hair pulling, lip or nail-biting)
- ☐ Powerful or sudden food cravings, constant hunger or loss of appetite
- ☐ Difficulty feeling satisfied while eating, regularly eating until over-full or uncomfortable
- ☐ Digestive distress (gas, bloating, stomach pain, constipation or diarrhea, irritable bowel)
- ☐ Carpal tunnel syndrome, tendon soreness
- ☐ Swollen or inflamed joints
- ☐ Loss of libido or marked lack of interest in sensual contact
- ☐ Frequent colds and infections
- ☐ Asthma or wheezing
- ☐ Elevated cholesterol, blood pressure, or c-reactive protein
- ☐ Blood sugar and insulin imbalances

__ Total Boxes Checked (of 42)

You might consider doing this review at the beginning of the the Healthy Deviant Adventure program, and then again a few months later.

I'm not suggesting that you'll see dramatic improvements in all (or even any) of your symptoms during the span of the program. But it can be helpful to stay aware of them, and to relay to your body that you are tracking them, interested in them, willing to make resolving them a priority.

And it may very well be that you *do* notice some differences. If so, note them on your Daily Deviance Journal Pages or Healthy Deviant Adventure Tracker.

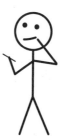

Learning to Love Your List

How did you do with the Weird Symptom Checklist? If you checked zero boxes, rock on. I hope it stays that way. But if you checked a bunch (or thought of some additional, unlisted symptoms that you *could* have checked), don't be too surprised. Twenty years ago, I would have checked almost all of them, and in my more depleted moments, I still check a few now and then.

Particularly if you think of yourself as pretty healthy, it can be alarming to go through a list like this and realize how many little (and not so little) things might be "wrong with you." But there's another way to look at it. Maybe these weird symptoms, while unpleasant and disconcerting, are not wrong and bad; maybe they are appropriate and potentially helpful reflections of what's going on in your body, your mind, and your life—and what could be going better. Seen this way, your symptoms are not your enemies, but your friends.

I know, this is not the way we're taught to think about our health, but this is another important Healthy Deviant perspective-shift worth considering. Because if you accept the "normal" view ("Symptoms are the enemy! Just make them go away!"), you're going to be putting yourself at a huge health disadvantage. Here's why: Many of the conditions we now consider "chronic diseases" reliably progress from symptoms like these—symptoms that are functional indicators of bodies and lives out of balance. But our conventional medical system isn't set up to deal with bodies and lives out of balance. It's set up to fix acute traumas and infectious diseases. Accordingly, it tends to ignore or suppress subtle-but-escalating symptoms until they converge to meet the definition of an official "differential" diagnosis.

This represents a potentially deadly waiting game. You persist in a state of "subclinical" declining health for months or years until one day, your lab numbers get bad enough or your symptoms severe enough and, presto—you now meet the standards of an official diagnosis profile. Congrats, you are the proud new owner of a bona fide disease! Once you have an official name for your disease, there are officially designated treatments. Most are limited to more symptom-suppressing drugs and perhaps some surgical interventions. Few address the underlying causes and root imbalances that gave rise to your disease in the first place.

This approach virtually guarantees that lifestyle-related diseases won't be addressed at the early stages, when they are most easily prevented and reversed. It also guarantees that most people who are suffering from them will never get better (even if their symptoms are temporarily forced into submission). On the contrary, if their current lifestyle habits and conditions persist, they are much more likely to get *worse*, racking up new diagnoses and new prescriptions and bigger medical bills as the years go by.

But I don't want you (or anyone) to suffer the current fate of "most people." That's why I'm a big fan of looking at your symptoms as helpful early-warning indicators of bigger troubles that could be coming down the pike. They are the check-engine lights on your body's dashboard. Busting them or putting duct tape over them makes no sense. Your symptoms are trying to tell you that something's going funky (see "Pissed-Off Body Syndrome," below), and if you listen closely, they will often tell you how to put it right.

Here's another way to think about it. A symptom is like a message in a bottle, a message meant for you. You can read your message now or toss it back out to sea for a while. Eventually, though, it will come back in on a bigger wave, accompanied by more bottles. You can ignore the accumulating collection of bottles bobbing on your shore for as long as you like—until they eventually come in on even bigger waves, first drenching you, then knocking you down, and eventually pulling you under.

By the time most people are sixty, they've got a whole lot of bottles washing up. And they are taking an average of *five* prescription drugs daily. All of which makes me wonder how much of what we think of as "aging" is really just the predictable result of unrepaired damage and delayed maintenance that has been going on for decades. I invite you to ponder that a moment, then look at your checklist again, seeing your checked boxes through new eyes. If you can't yet "love" your annoying and worrisome symptoms (and I get that!), just hold them in a neutral space for now.

When you read my story, and reflect a bit more on your own, I think you'll have a better understanding why at least *respecting* your symptoms is such an important part of the Healthy Deviant approach.

Pissed-Off Body Syndrome

Pissed-Off Body Syndrome describes a broad category of conditions and chronic diseases that emerge when the body is not happy about some aspect of the way we are living. The body then does its level best to let us know that by throwing up all sorts of symptoms and flares.

Pissed-Off Body Syndrome, as I define it, comprises most of the ailments that currently send people to doctors' offices and clinics in search of relief. These include fatigue, chronic pain, migraines and headaches of all sorts, digestive distress, ulcers, irritable bowel, acne, psoriasis, eczema, rashes, hormone imbalances, depression, overuse injuries, low back pain, joint swelling, and more.

It also includes a lot of the annoying symptoms, problematic lab results, and "off" feelings we have long before those more dramatic problems emerge.

Many mysterious, complex diseases with fancy sounding names (including, I suspect, a great many diseases that have "no known cause" and for which conventional treatments are not terribly effective) are all basically just some version of Pissed-Off Body Syndrome. That includes a lot of the problems you'll see in the "Weird Symptom Checklist," above.

The only way to cure Pissed-Off Body Syndrome is to figure out what is pissing the body off, and then stop doing that.

The problem is, most conventional doctors are not very good at recognizing the root causes of Pissed-Off Body Syndrome, much less at helping you to reverse it. There are reasons for that:

- It is not a topic taught in medical school (which is too bad, given that 97.3 percent of American adults are evidently suffering from it or will be soon).

- It doesn't have an official ICD (medical diagnostic code) or CPT (medical billing code).

- It is not something for which a doctor can confidently prescribe an approved pharmaceutical drug or medical procedure.

- It is a syndrome from which most medical doctors are themselves suffering.

- It is so pervasive that it has now become the normal state of most humans in our society.

You run a real risk of contracting Pissed-Off Body Syndrome whenever the body doesn't like something you are putting into it or on it, doing to it, asking of it, or otherwise exposing it to. It typically results from protracted states of irritation, imbalance, inflammation, toxicity, overload, and dozens of other assaults from the Unhealthy Default Reality.

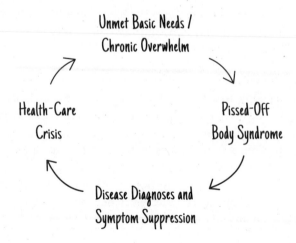

Unmet Basic Needs / Chronic Overwhelm

Pissed-Off Body Syndrome

Disease Diagnoses and Symptom Suppression

Health-Care Crisis

Pissed-Off Body Syndrome is often triggered by some combination of unmet needs and overwhelming demands. That includes eating an imbalanced or low-nutrition diet; eating or drinking things you are intolerant of or that damage your intestinal lining; not drinking enough water; exposure to toxic ingredients, chemicals, or environments; from not moving your body enough; elevated stress levels; sleep deficits; overrunning your available resources and energy; excessive stimuli or anxiety; and lack of meaning, connection, pleasure, social support, love, affection, and joy.

Pissed-Off Body Syndrome can be triggered into high gear by a trauma, major stress, or any dramatic life event. And it is generally exacerbated by the ongoing lack of respect, attention, and repair opportunities we offer our bodies while under the Unhealthy Default Reality's sway.

It other words, Pissed-Off Body Syndrome is the natural outcome of living in the Unhealthy Default Reality. And the only way to cure it is to remove, avoid, or actively compensate for the irritating, overwhelming, and undermining factors that are giving rise to it.

Doing that requires Healthy Deviance. And because Healthy Deviance flies in the face of the Unhealthy Default Reality and demands resources it is currently absorbing, resolving Pissed-Off Body Syndrome generally requires you to actively reclaim and redirect some part of those drained resources (especially your energy, attention, and mojo) for the express purpose of returning yourself to health.

Bottom line: You cannot cure Pissed-Off Body Syndrome while continuing to piss off your body.

Keep in mind, though, that the Unhealthy Default Reality will never teach you anything that will move you beyond Pissed-Off Body Syndrome. You have to do that for yourself. You do this by meeting your body-mind's unmet needs, and either reducing your overwhelm or finding ways to rise above it.

You can begin any time you like. Your body will begin healing, and forgiving, from the moment you start.[29]

Requisite legal disclaimer: I am not a medical doctor and my Weird Syndrome Checklist is not intended to diagnose or treat any condition or disease. Pissed-Off Body Syndrome is not a medically recognized condition. It is just a term I made up as a novel way of thinking about the health challenges a lot of us are having. If you have any health concerns that you think might require the attention of a medical doctor or other health professional, please consult one without delay.

Love the Body You're In

You know what? Most of us could stand to be a lot nicer to our bodies. And our bodies could do with a whole lot less hostility.

Even if you are currently suffering in your body, even if you are inherently unsatisfied with its present condition or downright angry with it for letting you down in some way, it can help to recognize that your body is, under the circumstances, serving you to the very best of its ability. It can also help to entertain the notion that your body might very well be reflecting its displeasure with how *you* are treating *it*.

Could you start a positive conversation with your body? Could you befriend it, and establish an open, respectful relationship that does your whole-person system good? My friend Jacquelyn Fletcher (JacquelynFletcher.com) has written a whole series of beautiful "Dear You" books in which she articulates the thoughts and feelings that have come up as she has related with her own body-mind, and ultimately healed that relationship at a deep level.

You might try writing your body a "Dear You" letter of your own, perhaps starting with a word of apology for the ways you've been out of touch or unkind. From there, share your gratitude that your body has stuck with you this long. Tell it about the relationship you would *like* to have. Ask your body what it would like you to know, and perhaps do differently. Then listen.

Wounded-Core Syndrome: Healing Trauma

If, in listening to your body, you hear from inner whisperings about adverse childhood events (ACEs) or trauma of any kind, get some help following that trail, because for many, unhealed traumas and post-traumatic stress are the unidentified root causes of numerous health challenges and increased disease risks.

For deeper reading on this topic, I recommend the work of psychiatrist James Gordon, MD, founder of the Center for Mind Body Medicine. He is an internationally recognized expert in the art of helping people reverse the psychological and biological damage done by all sorts of devastating losses and violent experiences, including population-wide traumatic events. Check out his most recent book, *The Transformation: Discovering Healing and Wholeness After Trauma.*

I also highly recommend the work of Resmaa Menakem, MSW, LICSW, SEP, author of *My Grandmother's Hands: Racialized Trauma and the Pathway to Mending Our Hearts and Bodies.* Menakem, a therapist who served for two years as a military contractor in Afghanistan, addresses both racialized and ancestral trauma (from which, he notes, we *all* suffer) in a particularly wise, compassionate, and embodied way. If you want a sense of Menakem's wisdom, listen to the podcast episode I recorded with him for *The Living Experiment* (titled "Trauma 1") at LivingExperiment.com and learn more about his work (including his free online course) at Resmaa.com.

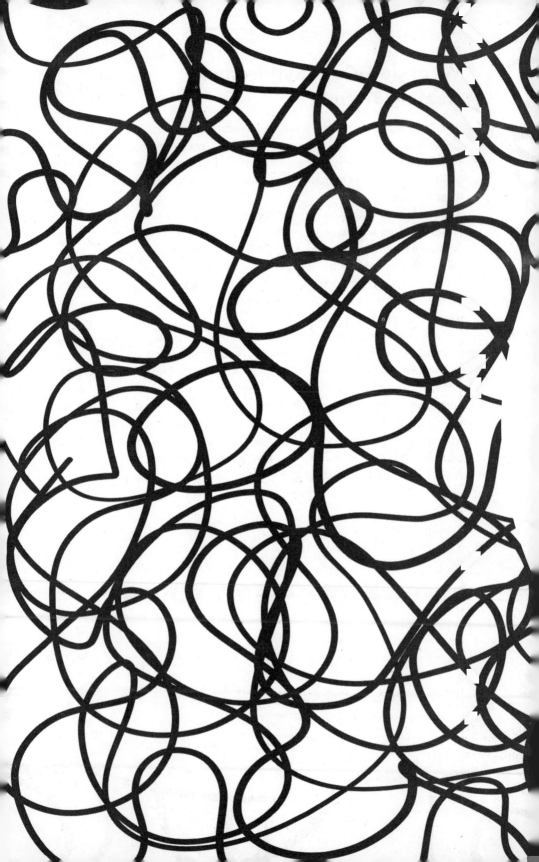

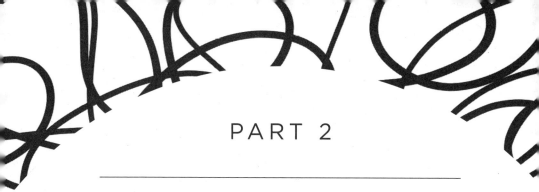

PART 2

The Making of a Healthy Deviant

(My Story—and Yours)

We shall not cease from exploration,
and the end of all our exploring will be to arrive
where we started and know the place for the first time.
—T. S. ELIOT

In the Beginning

No matter what happens,
it is within my power
to turn it to my advantage.

—EPICTETUS

My own journey to becoming a healthy and happy person is, in essence, a riches-to-rags-to-riches story. I started off as a pretty healthy kid. I got unhealthy. I figured stuff out, and I got better. Yay! The end.

I'm guessing you've read some version of that happy-ending story a million times. And if that's all you need to know about me for now, you can move happily on to the next chapter. But if you want my *real* story, the true story, you must know that it's more complicated, more nuanced. Like so much that is true (including your own story), it can't easily be reduced to a neat little headline or pat makeover story.

My real story is that I grew up with unconventional parents in unconventional times. I had an unconventional upbringing, and an unconventional education. I had some extraordinary advantages. *And still* ... none of that spared me walking the same conventional, downward-spiral path that the vast majority of people in our culture do. Like many young people, I didn't really want to be different. I wanted to be special and admired, sure, but I didn't want to be *weird*. That story has everything to do with how I got into trouble, and also with how I got out of it. In truth, I think a lot of the most important parts of our stories are a lot alike.

We all come into this world essentially who and how we are—small animals equipped to navigate toward adulthood. We are formed by all we observe, all we experience, all we ingest. And so we gradually become who we are today, loaded with beliefs and perceptions, preferences, and predilections. We build the skills and aptitudes necessary to survive in the world that presents itself to us. And we learn to present ourselves to it in the ways we believe will help us survive.

In our initial, natural state, our brains are so plastic and so fast-expanding that our pace of learning is almost impossible to conceive. A lot of that learning is dedicated to understanding our physical world and where we fit into it.

Little by little, first at home and then at school, we are taught where we begin and end. We are taught how things work and what we need to do to get by. We learn what is ours and not ours. We learn to sit in chairs and color inside of lines. We learn what is considered "good," "attractive," and "normal." We learn to compare ourselves with others. We learn to watch television, to operate electronic devices, to make and spend money. We learn who is in control, whose opinions and decisions count most, and who has a right to boss other people around. We learn what we're supposed to want, what we're supposed to dread, and what we're supposed to be ashamed of.

Slowly but surely, we go through the process of becoming civilized and indoctrinated into modern society. We become enmeshed with and subsumed by the Unhealthy Default Reality. We go from being a small animal equipped to make sense of the natural world, our own experience, and our own small, intimate social unit, to being an adult whose priorities are largely determined by mass media, complex social hierarchies, and large institutions. We spend the rest of our lives trying to navigate in ways that balance our basic human needs with the agendas set for us by the outside world. Our natural appetites, energy patterns, and priorities all shift accordingly.

Somewhere, beneath the conditioning and programming that the Unhealthy Default Reality imposes on us, the DNA of that original small animal still exists. The essential operating instructions and central nervous system remain much as they were when we came into the world. Our natural state is still accessible to us if we choose to access it.

This is not something the Unhealthy Default Reality teaches us. It's something we must discover for ourselves. We discover it, often, through what I call the Healthy Deviant Hero's Journey. Each version of that journey is unique, but they all have something in common: the unlearning of at least some of what the Unhealthy Default Reality has taught us, and the rediscovery of at least some remnants of our natural state.

That is a big part of why I am sharing some parts of my own Healthy Deviant Hero's Journey with you here. My goal here is not to bore you with the details of my personal experience; it is to help you zero in on the details of your own. It is also to help you understand that a great deal of the worthwhile wisdom I hope to impart in this book comes from having learned things the hard way.

I don't know about you, but whenever I meet people who know things, I want to know how they came to know them. Not just the books they read or the studies they completed, but the essence of what they have lived and learned for themselves. My own story says a lot about how I know what I know—not just in my brain, but also in my flesh and bones, in my heart. So I will share that story with you here.

I also want to ask you about *your* story. So, as I walk you though my own journey, I'll be offering you some questions and points of awareness to consider about your own life experiences, and the social and cultural influences that have shaped them. Because what you experienced up until this point has a lot to do with how things are for you now. I think reflecting on that may powerfully shape what you decide to do next.

The Healthy Deviant Hero's Journey

One thing the Unhealthy Default Reality does with great efficiency is convince us that we are inadequate failures and that we should expend all our energy and resources striving to become something that the Unhealthy Default Reality can accept and approve of.

That experience plays out differently for each of us, but with some surprisingly similar results: stress, anxiety, insecurity, and struggle. Fortunately, if you stay the course, the experience takes a turn at some point, and for most of us, it winds up imparting some surprisingly consistent gifts: insight, skill, empowerment, and a sense of purpose.

What I've noticed is that for a great many of us, this experience goes something like a hero's journey—that mythic, universal tale that Joseph Campbell describes in his classic book *The Hero with a Thousand Faces*.

The Healthy Deviant Hero's Journey, as I see it, depicts a story of formation that originates with one's natural state, proceeds through a series of trials and formative experiences, and then evolves to toward a self-possessed state of Healthy Deviance.

Healthy Deviant Hero's Journey

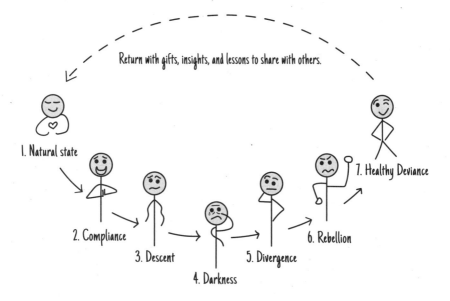

Here's an overview of how those different stages tend to proceed:

 Natural State: This is our entry point into the world, and into ourselves. Barring birth traumas or congenital challenges, we typically arrive in a reasonably healthy condition, comfortable in our own skin, unashamed, curious, and open to the world around us, eager to discover all that is within our reach. In this state, we feel like part of a larger whole, with nothing to prove and no need to earn outside approval. We take pleasure in simply being and in feeling connected to all that surrounds us.

Compliance: Here we begin registering and conforming to social expectations and norms. Adopting and internalizing our society's preferences, we invest increasing amounts of energy in trying to "fit in" or perform the roles we are told that we must. We strive to live up to the ideals and images that are presented to us as "normal" and desirable. We start to notice the ways that we don't measure up. We fear judgment and exclusion on the basis of our points of difference or perceived inadequacy. The goal of "good enough" seems forever beyond reach. We try to purchase, practice, and attain our society's markers of success. Or, in some cases, we simply try to survive.

Descent: Here we experience the building sense of stress, anxiety, insecurity, and impending failure that comes up from struggling to comply with unachievable standards or to endure intolerable pain. Our health and happiness degrade as the result of stress, strain, self-denial, and counterproductive interventions. Our energy, vitality, self-confidence, and self-regard are all depleted through our efforts at self-improvement, self-correction, or self-soothing. In our increasing urgency to fix whatever we see as "wrong with us" and to have or achieve what we are told will make us happy, we may become increasingly dependent on outside agents and experts to tell us what to do, or at least to find us acceptable.

 Darkness: Struggling and suffering with a growing assortment of unconscious behaviors and compulsive coping mechanisms, we feel a deepening sense of helplessness, hopelessness, and desperation. We may experience a severe dissatisfaction with our appearance, achievements, and place in the world, and we may be increasingly alienated from our own body. Feeling out of control, victimized, and emotionally reactive, we may be frequently anxious, depressed, tearful, rageful, reactive, critical, or withdrawn. We may be inclined to seeking oblivion or anesthesia through drugs, alcohol, food, sex, gambling, digital distraction, risk-taking, or other self-numbing, self-distracting, or self-soothing dependencies.

 Divergence: Approaching or arriving at an unsustainable, rock-bottom state, we decide that we don't want to (or can't) keep living the way we have been. Moving away from conventional improvement prescriptions and interventions, we may seek other forms of professional help or spiritual guidance, and new sources of social support. As we begin breaking away from the status quo, we may pursue more progressive forms of health care (such as alternative, integrative, and functional medicine) and more progressive forms of personal exploration. We may experiment with new ways of eating, moving, or living. Discovering that a lot of what works for us is *not at all what we've been told to do,* and also not what most other people are doing, we start to care less whether other people understand or approve of our choices. We decide that the rewards of our difference are greater than the costs.

 Rebellion: Striking out on our own path toward health, we may look to other Healthy Deviants for counsel and perspective. In this stage, we may feel relieved to have discovered approaches that are actually working, but also angry, resentful, or mortified about all that we've been put through (or put ourselves through) on the way to this better place. We may be outraged or dumbfounded that nobody has told us there are easier, better, more effective ways to approach health and happiness. We may regret having wasted so much time, money, and energy on things that don't work. Feeling that we've suffered unjustly, we may be given to railing against the oppressive, conspiratorial forces of the Unhealthy Default Reality, including mass media, mass health care, big food, big oil, big pharma, the government, the patriarchy, the military industrial complex, colonialism, and more. Uncertain whom to blame, we may find ourselves waving our fists in the air at all the powers that be.

 Healthy Deviance: Realizing that while rebellion can be a useful and necessary state, it can also be exhausting and negative-minded, we begin seeking a more sustainable and enjoyable position to play from. In this stage, we begin to recognize that through all our trials and tribulations, we have become stronger, wiser, better versions of ourselves. Feeling grateful for our own hard-won knowledge and experience, and relieved that life no longer seems as hard, we feel a growing desire to give back. Knowing that we carry insights and gifts that others can benefit from, we long to share them with anyone who wants to learn. We get comfortable with the fact that even though we've arrived in a better place, we will inevitably step back and forth between all the positions on the Healthy Deviant Hero's Journey. Sometimes we will inhabit more than one spot—or hold the viewpoints of more than one station—simultaneously.

The Return: Consistent with a classic hero's journey, the final stage of the Healthy Deviant Hero's Journey represents a "return" phase. Because at this point, all of the stages of our journey live within us, we now have the opportunity to reinhabit the easy, authentic, natural state that is our birthright. We no longer feel we have something to fix or prove, but rather, that we are here to witness and observe with empathy, to do some good, to relieve unnecessary waste and suffering. We now carry wisdom, resources, and inspiration—the bounty gathered on all the previous stages of our voyage—and feel compelled to share them with others. This can manifest as a "pay it forward" instinct focused on helping individuals struggling with our former challenges or as a generalized passion for making positive change in the wider world.

Here's how those phases played out for me … and what I wonder about how they've played out for you.

6

Act 1: Natural State

You do not have to be good. You do not have to walk on your knees for a hundred miles through the desert, repenting. You only have to let the soft animal of your body love what it loves.

—MARY OLIVER

My Story

I was born in 1967. It was the winter just before the Summer of Love—which was also the summer of urban race riots. The *Mad Men* era was fading. Civil rights and Vietnam War protests were in full swing. The Apollo Space Program was underway. The Beatles, the Rolling Stones, Aretha Franklin, and Jimi Hendrix were rocking people's worlds.

In reaction to the conservative, hyper-conformity of the 1950s and early 1960s, the late 1960s and early 1970s were all about counterculture rebellion, exploration, and experimentation. Established boundaries and assumptions were being openly challenged. Society was grappling with discordant mores and manners, confronting the oppression of women and people of color, rethinking ideologies that had produced war, poverty, segregation, and inequality. As a result, many people were actively reconsidering what "normal" meant, and feeling less and less constrained by that definition. Younger folks grew their hair long and rejected the more conservative values of their parents.

My parents, though, were not conservative. On the contrary, they were super progressive. My mother was a young, back-to-the-land, earth-mother type. My dad was a sociologist who saw social norms as culturally variable and historically shifting constructs. Neither cared much for convention. So I was brought up as a flower child, and as a baby, I was pretty much encouraged to be my natural baby self.

My earliest memories are of regarding the world around me with pleasure and fascination. The most vivid of those memories is of a particular day when I was swinging in a tire swing that was tied to a high branch of a tree in our yard. I was probably about two. I remember I was wearing little red shoes and looking out over them as I swung, seeing the bright red leather pass over the green of the grass, the blue of the sky, and then the white of the clouds. I was at peace in myself in that moment, content with my relationship to the world. This is as close as I can recall to being in what I now call my natural state.

Your Story

Reflecting back as far as you can, can you recall a memory from any part of your childhood (or later life) in which you felt completely at peace and okay in your body? A moment when you felt unselfconscious but aware, connected with the world around you, but also clear on your own individuality?

See if you can find even a tiny memory like that, and describe it in careful detail. It does not need to be an outwardly significant moment, but it will probably be a moment in which you can describe with some precision the sensory experience of being in your body.

If you can't recall a particular moment, just picture yourself as an infant, coming fresh into the world, emerging directly from nature's most basic processes, without any sense that you should be anything other than what you are. Sit with that feeling a moment, and see if you can tap back into the experience of being in the right time at the right place without anything to prove or produce. See if you can access the feeling of being some whole, simple, unadulterated version of yourself.

Reflect for a moment on these areas of inquiry, and if you like, note your answers in a journal.

Act 2: Compliance

Until they become conscious they will never rebel and
until after they have rebelled they cannot become conscious.

—GEORGE ORWELL, *1984*

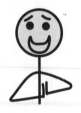

The era of my early childhood was, in some ways, a period not unlike the one we find ourselves in now: Polarizing, intense, fluid, full of surprises and rapid changes—not all of them easy to grapple with. During the time of my toddlerhood, a new interest in Eastern and esoteric philosophy, spirituality, and yoga emerged. Sexual prohibitions were relaxed. Psychedelic drugs and marijuana were embraced. Many followed Timothy Leary's advice to "turn on, tune in, and drop out."

College campuses across the country became epicenters not only for huge peace and civil-rights protests but also for a great deal of new intellectual thought, social experimentation, and personal exploration. This was a time when academic subjects and classroom practices were struggling to keep pace with the times.

It was a dynamic, disruptive moment for the social sciences, in particular—fields like sociology, anthropology, psychology—because they were tasked not just with interpreting and explaining the unprecedented goings on, but also with charting a course to a better reality.

The human-potential movement was picking up steam. The field known as positive psychology (which focuses on nurturing positive traits and optimal experiences rather than studying pathological behavior and neuroses) was just taking nascent form.

Throughout my early childhood, my dad taught in the sociology department at Lake Forest College in Illinois. While acting as chair of the department, he hired a promising young psychology professor, Mihaly Csikszentmihalyi, to come work with him. My dad knew Csikszentmihalyi—now famous for his seminal work on flow states ("the psychology of optimal experience") from the University of Chicago, where they had done postgraduate coursework together.

Collaborating with other faculty and students, they explored new concepts in what it meant to be human, to accept or depart from constraining social norms, to be authentic, self-examined, and fully realized as an individual within a supportive community—or alternatively, to be oppressed by limiting beliefs, discrimination, dogma, and the strictures of a dominant society.

Our house became a gathering place for progressive thinkers. Long, rambling conversations took place around our dinner table. Debates ensued in our living room. In our backyard, over jugs of red wine, intellectual arguments were bandied about. Social constructs were reconsidered. Old philosophies were argued, new ideas examined.

Before he earned his doctorate, my father (a first-generation Greek American) had worked his way through school digging ditches, washing dishes, and operating cranes in the steel mills of Gary, Indiana. He was forever asking questions like, "Why do we live the way we live? How does our society shape and limit our choices and assumptions? How do our cultural mores and manners encourage or prohibit the development of the best within us?"

My mother, meanwhile, was inclined to ask a different set of questions, like, "How can we make the world more the way we would *like* it to be? How can we opt out of those structures and strictures that aren't in our best collective interest, and create new, more rewarding models of our own?" She had grown up on a Midwestern farm and always felt a strong connection with nature, art, and spirituality. As she grew up, she morphed from a free-wheeling farm tomboy to feminist-hippie utopian idealist. She did yoga, joined a food co-op, made organic whole-grain bread and bean sprouts, listened to Joni Mitchell, and studied the I Ching.

Like many young women of her era, my mother questioned the gender-based prescriptions of her society. While she enjoyed being a mom, she felt straight-jacketed by the social expectations around her roles as homemaker and faculty wife. Still in her late twenties and just discovering herself as an individual, my mom began attending consciousness-raising women's groups with her best friend (and fellow faculty wife), Mary Ellen. Together, they began making plans to start a back-to-the-land communal farm where they could raise their kids in the context of a cooperative community.

In the early 1970s, my mom convinced my dad that the family should move to Minnesota, where she'd grown up. My dad took a job at a small liberal arts college in the heart of Minneapolis. Most weekends, while Dad was grading papers, Mom and Mary Ellen roamed the rural countryside, looking for the farm of their dreams. On one of their jaunts, they found it—a dilapidated 250-acre property in Wisconsin. With money pooled from parents and siblings, they purchased it.

For the next few years, with lots of help from relatives, friends, and various passers-through, they set about making the farm livable. They cleaned up junked cars and tore down old buildings, salvaging the materials to build new ones. They planted hay and grain; raised cows, pigs, and chickens; and grew huge vegetable gardens for food. It was an immense undertaking. But they had a vision: A thriving community where they could create a good, simple, satisfying life by living in harmony with nature and each other.

We started out spending our summers at the farm. In retrospect, it was about the healthiest upbringing any child could hope for. Plenty of fresh air, sunshine, and physical activity; lots of nutritious, homegrown organic food; no television (video games, cell phones, laptops, and iPads hadn't even been invented yet); endless opportunities for creative play; living in accordance with natural daily cycles and seasonal rhythms.

It sounds great. And in many ways, it was. But it wasn't always easy—for us *or* our parents. As happens in many intentional communities, there was a regular stream of discord over everything from gardening and child-rearing styles to romantic jealousies and financial priorities. It took a toll on my parents' marriage. When I was about eight, they decided to separate. Remaining friendly, they agreed on joint custody. My dad would remain in the city, and my mom would move to the farm full time. My sisters and I could live where we liked and go back and forth as we pleased.

Through grade school, we opted to live with Mom at the farm, attending a local three-room schoolhouse during the week, and spending weekends in the city with Dad. As we reached high school age, we moved to live with him full time, in part because the schools in the Twin Cities were better, and in part because we were ready for a change of pace. For me, at least, the farm had just started feeling a little too insular, a little too ... weird.

As I had matured from childhood to adolescence, I had begun to understand that our communal farm was an unconventional place, that we were living in a very unconventional way. And increasingly, that made me uncomfortable. Like most kids my age, I just wanted to fit in.

I was forever asking my mom questions like, "Why do we have to bring this weird homemade bread for lunch? How come my sandwich has watercress on it? Why don't we have Cheetos, Fritos, and Twinkies like the other kids have? And why don't you wear a bra or at least put on some lipstick?"

Similarly, I often complained to my father, "Why do you always have to question everything that society says is good and normal? What is the point of criticizing what everybody else seems to think is fine? How am I supposed to make friends if I'm always acting different from everyone else? And why can't you dress like a regular professor?"

By the time I was ten, I was concerned that the "normal" world was passing me by. Disco was happening, lip gloss, diet soda, and designer jeans were happening. I felt certain I was missing out. My wholesome, counterculture childhood had led me to dread being seen as "different." I didn't want to live on some weird organic farm for the rest of my life. I wanted to live in the *real* world. I wanted to be *normal*. So at twelve, I left the farm behind and went to live in the city with my dad. Meanwhile, like many kids, I tried hard to forget everything my parents had taught me.

Your story: Consider your childhood. What were you were taught (by lesson or example) to see as normal or abnormal, healthy or unhealthy, desirable or disgusting? What was the social and historical context of your upbringing? What trends and events were you and your family influenced by? When and how did your first health challenges emerge, and how they were dealt with?

Areas for review: Early health influences and role models. Memorable images and media messaging. Significant events or traumas. Patterned behaviors and routines. Your earliest memories about your relationship with your body. The ways you learned to conform with (and/or resist) social and cultural expectations.

Reflect for a moment on these areas of inquiry, and if you like, note your answers in a journal.

Act 3: Descent

In a mad world, only the mad are sane.

—AKIRA KUROSAWA

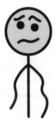

In about 1980, when I began living with my father and sisters in Minneapolis, I experienced an abrupt shift in lifestyle. My newly single working dad didn't really have time or inclination to cook. So while he did his best to feed us decent meals, we were often left to our own devices. Even though we generally had fresh vegetables and fruits in the house, most everything I chose to eat came from a can, bag, or box.

Living with our mom at the farm throughout the 1970s, we'd been sheltered from a lot of the changes that had been taking place in the U.S. food supply. During that time, processed and convenience foods had proliferated wildly.

Fast foods had gone from being an occasional treat to a regular source of sustenance for many busy families. After a childhood of bean sprouts, beef tongue, goat's milk, and carob cookies, my sisters and I were just fine with this. *Finally, some normal stuff!*

My dad wouldn't let us have sugary cereals or soft drinks in the house, but he'd let us have Cheerios and Grape-Nuts (which we'd eat from giant bowls with lots of added sugar when he wasn't looking). And on the nights he was working, we'd have Lean Cuisine TV dinners or order pizza.

In our new urban environment, there weren't nearly as many opportunities to be active or to spend time outside. So when we weren't studying, we mostly watched television—something we'd had no access to at the farm.

As a sociologist, my dad always loved watching television. He enjoyed interpreting its cultural messages. With an academic's detachment, he delighted in its ironies, its absurdity, its unabashed sensationalism.

He would often grade exams or pay bills in front of a tiny black-and-white television set in our living room. Periodically, he would call us over to come see this or that phenomenon of interest: An evangelist publicly admitting to cheating on his wife, game show contestants going berserk over being called to "come on down," advertisements with inherently discriminatory imagery or hyper-consumerist messages, amusingly melodramatic soap operas.

"Incredible," my dad would say, grinning and shaking his head. "Can you *believe* this stuff?" For him, it was all great fodder for his college courses, many of which revolved around getting his students to begin seeing their society through the objective, critical eyes of a social explorer.

Although I didn't realize it at the time, this way of looking at the world would make an immense (albeit delayed) impact on my perceptions, giving me a strange knack for simultaneously participating in and curiously observing the world around me. I now consider this sort of social observation an essential healthy-person skill. But at the time, I just thought my dad was eccentric—particularly when he summoned all of us to gather around the screen: "Hey kids! Come in here! You gotta see this!"

Mostly, he called us to come see the craziness and dysfunction that was modern mass culture. But occasionally we'd get the call to come take in some great scene from a vintage or foreign film he loved. Sometimes, we watched together just for fun. It was a way we bonded as a family, a way we created coziness.

Being an anxious introvert, I started watching a lot of television when I was alone, too. As I moved into my awkward teenage years, television become a dependency for me—a solace, a distraction, a place to hide out. As a result, despite my father's intellectual and ironic distance from it, television became an increasingly important influence on my ideology, attitudes, and sense of self. Game-show spokesmodels and talk-show celebrities; soap operas and sitcom characters—in my mind, all of them broadcast clear images of what I was supposed to look like, act like, live like, and be.

Between show segments, a stream of thirty-second ads dictated the list of products I'd need in order to have any hope of achieving those ideals: clothes, cosmetics, hair-care products, and diet aids. Meanwhile, the 1980s gave rise to an even greater variety of processed food products. Microwavable, snackable, and instant things flooded onto the market. So did low-fat diet foods and artificially sweetened beverages. Because by now, obesity rates were climbing fast.

When I was born, only about 10 percent of U.S. adults were considered overweight or obese. By the time I graduated from college, that number had doubled. As of today, it has nearly tripled.

You might think that having been raised the way I was, I'd have been immune to all these influences. Not so. Instead, it was my distinct impression during my teenage years that society was right, and that my counterculture parents were at least partially to blame for my obvious inadequacy. In some way, by virtue of their stubborn nonconformity, I felt they had set me up to fail.

It seemed to me that instead of teaching me about what I *actually* needed to know, they'd been filling my head with nonsense, pursuing their own counterculture fancies while misdirecting me about what it was going to take for me to succeed in the real world.

Neither of my parents cared much for material things. We didn't have much money. Our cars were rusty. Everything was hand-me-down or from the thrift store. I stubbornly tried to convince my mother we should start buying more store-bought food, more fashionable clothes. I tried to convince my dad that he should stop pointing out society's foibles and just get with the program of how things were.

Meanwhile, I got to work fitting in and measuring up myself. Thanks to all the junk food and television watching (not to mention puberty), by the time I was thirteen or fourteen, I'd gained a few pounds. In my mind, this was not good. Not good at all. Clearly, *something had to be done.*

I started reading every fashion and beauty magazine I could get my hands on. I pored over the articles. I obsessed over the pictures. I tried to figure out the formula for female success. Here's what I took away: To be wanted, to be successful, to be worthy, I needed to be attractive. To be attractive, I had to be fashionably slender, and that meant being on a diet. Constantly.

My father happened to be dating a very thin woman at the time. Looking back, I now suspect she was anorexic, but back then, I just thought she was glamorous. One day, concerned with the numbers I saw on the scale, I asked her for some weight-loss advice. She counseled me to start avoiding fats and to start counting calories. Avocados? No. Too high in fat and calories. Diet soda? Yes, that was a "free" food. I could have as much as I liked. "Eat less, exercise more," she advised, counseling me to wear ankle weights around the house to burn off extra calories.

Back on the farm, we hadn't worried about calories or fats or portion sizes. We just ate the homegrown, homemade whole food we were served, stopping when we were full or when the food ran out. But this woman ate in a highly tactical way. She selected, rationed, measured, and burned off her food with precision. She seemed to know what she was doing.

I remember once, when we were out for dinner as a family, I was standing next to her in line at the salad bar. I put some chickpeas on my salad, and she visibly flinched. She leaned over and whispered to me, "Hey, just so you know, every one of those things has 16 calories. I know they *look* healthy, but they're super fattening."

"Woah!" I said, "I didn't know that!" Suddenly self-conscious and ashamed, I shoved most of the chickpeas off my plate.

For me, this was the beginning of a period of disordered eating. I would go long stretches eating very little, then binge on saltines and fat-free pudding. I would walk for miles with weights on every appendage, then sit in front of the television for hours trying to distract myself from my own hunger.

I wrote frequently in my journal about how flawed and inadequate I felt. I made long lists of the improvements I needed to make to my appearance just to be "okay." It felt exhausting and overwhelming, like being endlessly at war with myself. I would check my body in the mirror a hundred times a day and from a dozen different angles, pinching and frowning at the parts I didn't like. With what little money I could scrape together working part-time at retail stores, I bought clothes that I hoped would camouflage the worst of my body's failings and cosmetics to try and "correct" my less-than-perfect facial features. Once, when I was about thirteen, I got caught shoplifting some press-on fake fingernails. I needed them to cover my own, which I'd nervously bitten into ragged stubs.

What happened to me at this point in my life is what happens to a lot of people for their *entire* lives (and as a white, cis, middle-class woman, I recognize that in retrospect, I had it easy): The more I embraced the norms of our society, and the more I went along with the ideals of the dominant culture, the less healthy and happy I got. Then I went to college, and it all got worse.

Your story: Consider your teenage and young-adult years. What was going on with your health, happiness, and self-perceptions during that time? In retrospect, what aspects of your upbringing now strike you as healthy or unhealthy? When did you first start making your own choices about food, activity, and other things that impacted your health? How did those decisions play out? To what extent were you led to believe that "being on a diet" or "burning calories" was important to being a good, disciplined, acceptable, or attractive person?

Areas for review: Your shifting patterns of eating, activity, sleep, and social connection. Your experiences of puberty, body image, and early sexuality. Diet, fitness, and other appearance-improvement interventions. Feelings of shame, fear, anger, or anxiety based on "difference," or not fitting in. The emergence or continuation of nervous habits. The influences of technology, social media, and mass media on your perceptions and life rhythms. The pressures you felt to conform, to achieve, or to impress; the pull you felt to discover and define yourself as an individual.

Reflect for a moment on these areas of inquiry, and if you like, note your answers in a journal.

9

Act 4: Darkness

In a dark time, the eye begins to see.

—THEODORE ROETHKE

My college years are still a bit of a blur to me. I remember studying hard, and I got good grades, but my academic achievement came at a high cost to my body-mind. I often read and wrote papers late into the night. The constant barrage of quizzes and exams gave me extreme anxiety.

I ate a lot of cafeteria food and drank a lot of coffee. Aside from walking back and forth between my dorm, my classes, and the library, I didn't get much exercise. I was always parked at one desk or another, head down, reading and scribbling and typing until my eyes hurt and my neck ached.

I loved what I was learning, but I felt I always had more to do than I could possibly do well. My perfectionism grew more pronounced. My inner critic, always vocal, took on a nasty, threatening tone. I had a lot of foreboding conversations with myself, during my college years, about what would happen if I didn't "perform up to expectations" or achieve the "academic success" I was told I was capable of. No matter how many 4.0s earned, every 3.5 left me feeling like a disappointment to myself and others. Meanwhile, my health and happiness steadily unraveled. I gained weight, I got depressed, and I started having skin problems.

In my senior year, I earned a Fulbright teaching assistantship—a postgraduate scholarship that allowed me to move to Paris and teach in a French middle school. By this time, I thought that perhaps I wanted to be a professor like my dad, but a few months of teaching made it clear that the classroom life was not for me.

With no access to friends or family (this was before cell phones, and even before home internet), and with no social support system to fall back on, I felt profoundly lonely and exposed. Living on a meager stipend in one of the most expensive cities in the world, I could barely afford the rent on my tiny ninety-square-foot *chambre de bonne* (no kitchen, no shower, a shared, non-plumbed "toilet" in the filthy hall). Between paychecks, I often ran out of money. I'd get by on bread and water, or occasionally go without food entirely for a day or two at a time.

Meanwhile, all that French bread wasn't doing me any favors. I was becoming increasingly ill from an as-yet-undiagnosed gluten intolerance, and what I now recognize as the telltale signs of intestinal permeability. My skin broke out in cystic acne. My face and body swelled. My stomach cramped. My back ached.

Finally, in the winter of '91, I wound up leaving my Fulbright post a few months early to come home and heal. Within weeks of returning, I got into a car accident that resulted in a neck injury. The chiropractor who treated my neck took note of my other health issues and wondered aloud whether I might have a sensitivity to gluten. When I told her that my dad had always been gluten-intolerant (even back in the 1950s when nobody had heard of such a thing), she said that this was a common genetic trait, and I should try avoiding the stuff entirely. She gave me a long list of foods to avoid.

I followed her counsel, and found it helped enormously. Within a few days, my skin began clearing, my digestive issues cleared up, my back stopped aching, and my mood improved. But still, I was faced with a vexing problem: The question of what to do with my life.

For years after college, I took job after job, trying to figure out what I was good at, what I enjoyed, what I could to do make a living. And all the while, I felt I was failing at everything. In my mid-twenties, I met a man I fell head over heels for, but he was mercurial and unreliable. Sometimes he seemed interested in me. Other times he wouldn't call for weeks. Naturally, I became obsessed with him, convinced that my happiness depended on our being together. My self-esteem hit an all-time low, and my health took an even greater nose-dive as a result.

Although I was no longer suffering from gluten-triggered inflammation, I felt like a stranger in my own body. I didn't like the way that I looked, and I figured that if this guy didn't like me, it was obviously because there was something *wrong with me*. I wasn't thin enough or attractive enough or athletic enough ... or something.

I decided I would do two things: (1) focus on my career; and (2) "get into shape." For the better part of five years, I read nothing but self-help books and health and fitness magazines. I tried every diet and workout I could find. They all left me hungry, peevish, and exhausted. I developed uncontrollable cravings for sugar, fat, and salt.

Typically, my cravings would hit toward the end of the day, and when they did, they sent me running to the fast-food drive through for burgers and fries, to the grocery store for ice cream, and to the gas station on the corner for chips. I felt like I had a split personality—one part of me tightly controlling my eating and "working on myself," and the other part of me sabotaging those efforts with astonishing power.

At some point in my late twenties, I decided to give up on dieting. I felt like I just didn't have the willpower, and it wasn't doing me any good. And the more nutrition books I read (especially books like *Know Your Fats* by lipids researcher Mary Enig, PhD), the more I was coming to understand that a lot of what I'd been taught to believe about the "calories in, calories out" model of weight loss was all wrong.

Then I read *Nourishing Traditions: The Cookbook That Challenges Politically Correct Nutrition and the Diet Dictocrats* by Sally Fallon, and discovered what became, for me, a whole new field of interest: ancestral nutrition. Rather than avoiding fats, I began seeking out more and better ones. Rather than trying to eat less junk, I began trying to eat more protein and vegetables—which, weirdly, made me crave less junk. Suddenly, I felt like I had a lot more energy to exercise. I took up jogging and yoga. My skin took on a healthy glow I hadn't seen since my childhood.

Meanwhile, after a decade of what my grandmother referred to as "dead-end jobs," I had somehow found my way into marketing and custom publishing, an industry where my writing and communication skills made sense. I got promoted a few times, and I started making better money. I got a better car, a better apartment, better clothes. But as my career kicked into high gear, my career stress did, too.

After a few years of working inside an agency, I struck out on my own as a freelance consultant, keeping the agency as a retainer client. One of the first projects they sent me was a magazine, and over the course of about a year, I discovered I had a knack for that —coming up with article ideas, researching, writing, editing.

In my early thirties, still unsure of what I wanted to be when I grew up, I decided that since I enjoyed working on magazines, and since health was the topic that interested me most, I should try making a magazine about that. I wrote up a forty-page creative blueprint for a whole-person healthy-living magazine and, working through another custom publishing company, pitched the idea to Life Time Fitness (then one of the leading health-club companies in the area).

Incredibly, they said yes. And so began the hardest work of my life. I found myself pulling all-nighters trying to make what seemed like an unrelenting torrent of deadlines, and bit by bit, despite my healthy eating and exercise routines, my body began breaking down.

I developed a nasty red, peeling rash on my face, which was pronounced by my doctor to be *perioral dermatitis* (that's the Latinate medicalese term for "rash around the mouth"—gee, thanks doc). My eyelashes started falling out. I developed night sweats, back pain, stomach pain, and carpal tunnel syndrome. I experienced unexpected crying jags. I started accumulating prescriptions. Creams for the rashes. Antacids for the stomach pain. Chinese herbs for the night sweats.

This was, keep in mind, while I was *editing a health and fitness magazine.*

To be fair, I was by this time doing a lot of things "right." I was eating a reasonably healthy whole-foods diet, drinking mostly water. I had laid off the junk food. I was steering clear of gluten. I had even established a solid exercise routine, including running, kettlebells, yoga, and calisthenics. But the level of stress I was sustaining was way too much for my body to bear. I wasn't taking breaks. I wasn't breathing deeply. I wasn't sleeping enough. I was overdriving my systems.

One day, I was at my desk, editing an article that had already gone through three rewrites. It was now badly behind schedule, and, as I saw it, still not close to good enough. My temper rose steadily as I tried to edit the piece toward "acceptability." My mental focus evaporated. I couldn't think straight. I'd planned to take a run by the river, but now there was no time for that.

I decided to work off my frustration by dashing up and down the stairs a few times. Four breathless flights later, heart pounding, I was no less irritated, no less behind schedule, and that damn article was still sitting there, needing hours more work.

"I don't have time for this!" I thought. Something had to give. I stood there for a moment, frantic, shaking and sweating on the stair landing. Then, in a fit of self-directed fury, I stomped my foot on the wooden boards, hard. Too hard. Something snapped: My fifth metatarsal bone.

In the same moment that I heard the bone in my foot break, I felt my entire physiology give way. Like a balloon inflated to the point of bursting, I felt the tension that had been building within me blast outward. The cracking sound was sickening. The pain was excruciating. I fell in a crumpled heap, sobbing.

Your story: Reflect on how your adult life has been going, and how your body has responded to the challenges you've faced. What health-improvement strategies are working for you, and which against? What habits, patterns, or behaviors are causing you to feel frustrated or helpless? Has your body ever refused to go along with the plans you've made for it? Have you ever injured or done damage to some part of yourself (physical, mental, emotional, or spiritual) by trying to force your body beyond its natural limits or warning signals? What is your current level of readiness to change?

Areas for review: The extent to which you've been "making things work," but breaking yourself down in the process. Feelings of doubt, discontent, or inadequacy. Overdrawing your energetic (and perhaps financial) accounts in an attempt to keep up with life's demands. Pushing the limits of your own sanity and cell tissue. Looking for help with emerging health problems, and getting saddled with dead-end diagnoses and symptom-suppressing pre-scription drugs instead. Growing frustrated or hopeless about your body. The cage-rattling stress of not feeling up to what so-called normal life is asking of you.

Reflect for a moment on these areas of inquiry, and if you like, note your answers in a journal.

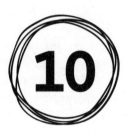

Act 5: Divergence

The thing that is really hard, and really amazing, is giving up on being perfect and beginning the work of becoming yourself.

—ANNA QUINDLEN

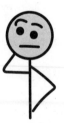

For a few minutes after I broke my foot, I sat there in shock, tears streaming down my face. Then I commando-crawled over to the phone, called my dad, and asked him to come take me to the emergency room. For the twenty minutes it took him to arrive, I lay there on the floor, thinking. And in that rare moment of reflection, of doing nothing, I had an aha moment. Three of them, actually:

- **First, I realized that I had literally just broken myself:** I had directed so much untethered violence against my own body that I had succeeded in snapping a piece of my own skeleton in two. That potential for self-violence both shocked and scared me.

- **Next, I realized (with some horror) that this was nothing new:** While this breaking of bone was novel, the larger dynamic of self-breakage was not. I had, in fact, *been* breaking myself—for years. I'd been breaking my digestion, my biochemistry, my brain, my hormones, my healthy limits, my self-regard.

- **Finally, I realized that I was not alone:** For as sorry as I might feel for myself in this crumpled-heap moment, when I thought about it, I had to acknowledge that pretty much everyone I knew was suffering from a similar set of symptoms and frustrations. And even though many were taking prescription medications to get by, most seemed to be getting worse, not better, over time.

And that is how, out of a moment of abject misery and self-pity came a moment of great clarity. The mass-media advice and popular health prescriptions I'd been attempting to follow simply were not working for me. Or for most of the people I knew. Period.

I got curious about why this was. And after a brief review of my own life history (amazing, the insights that can come to you while lying broken on the floor), I recognized that most of my health and fitness challenges were symptoms of a larger malady—namely, that I was chronically overwhelmed, overworked, overcritical, overstimulated, and overstressed. As a result, I was making reactive, half-conscious, self-sabotaging decisions most of the time.

The underlying problem, it seemed to me, was that I was living in a world where all the normal default choices were predominantly unhealthy choices. Most of the socially approved life patterns and habits were at total odds not just with my health but also with my very DNA.

No mere diet or exercise program was going to save me from this conundrum, I realized. Before I could make lasting changes to my eating and movement patterns, I had to first marshal enough awareness to responsibly steward both my energy and my attention in the midst of modern life. I had to reclaim responsibility for my own well-being, and that started with seeing and repairing the damage I'd done to myself over the previous three decades.

It didn't happen all at once, but slowly, bit by bit, I began letting go of a lot of conventional norms and health prescriptions in favor of doing what actually felt good to me. I reduced my intake of grain-based products and stopped avoiding fats, including saturated fats. Newly obsessed with the idea of phytonutrients, I started eating a much greater variety of vegetables, starting with breakfast.

I gave up bikini-body workouts and made a point of moving in ways I enjoyed. I embraced some primal-inspired exercise routines that worked a lot better for me than anything I had tried before. My energy improved. My body-composition shifted. I felt stronger, athletic even.

I gave up reading conventional health magazines and watching television. I began meditating, taking more breaks, listening to my body, allowing my mind to wander. I started spending more time outdoors each day, honoring my need for sleep, safeguarding time for play and relaxation. Suddenly, my life felt more doable. My problems less devastating. I started feeling ... hopeful.

I also stopped chasing the outward appearance of "success" as a metric of success. I began studying and experimenting with smarter, more satisfying ways to live and be. And as I experimented, something interesting happened. My life got incrementally better. Then dramatically better. I discovered that "normal" was indeed overrated—and also rather deadly, at least for me. I also discovered that there were a lot of alternatives I enjoyed more.

Your story: What catalysts, catastrophes or significant life events have triggered a reconsideration or meaningful change in how you approach your health and well-being? Have you experienced any rock-bottom moments or breaking points, and if so, have they brought you any significant insights or awarenesses? Can you see more such events on the horizon? What health trajectory have you been on, and what would it take for you to adjust that trajectory to your liking? What fears are holding you back?

Areas for review: The value of becoming your own rescuer. Safeguarding your sanity; building your capacity and skills. Dealing with doubt, criticism, disapproval, resistance, ridicule, and jealousy. Surrendering your attachment to being good enough, right, perfect, or even normal. Recognizing the ways you may be "breaking yourself." Working within your available means and known strengths. Discerning between real and fake role models; defining your own version of success.

Reflect for a moment on these areas of inquiry, and if you like, note your answers in a journal.

Act 6: Rebellion

Learning is always rebellion.... Every bit of new truth discovered
is revolutionary to what was believed before.

—MARGARET LEE RUNBECK

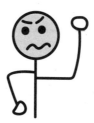

For a long time after I started figuring out what it actually took for me to be healthy in body and mind, I felt outraged that nobody had ever explained this to me before. A lot of what I was learning now was from weighty books, research papers, classes, and street-wise, deeply experienced healthy people. A lot of it was entirely different than what I'd learned from health and fitness magazines.

Frankly, a lot of what I was learning were lessons that my parents, bless them, had tried to impart when I was younger and disinclined to listen to anything they had to say. Somehow, even though I'd heard much of it before, studying and discovering it all for myself and from this new frame of mind made all the difference.

I learned about the food supply, and it entirely changed my perspective on groceries. I learned how food works like information, not just fuel, and it entirely changed the things I was hungry for. I learned about ancestral nutrition, traditional fats, organ meats, and bone-based nutrients, and it entirely shifted what I thought sounded appetizing.

I learned about how my cardiovascular system and muscles and joints worked, and it entirely changed my approach to movement, posture, breathing, and exercise. I learned about my DNA, my cells, my brain, my sympathetic and parasympathetic nervous systems, and it entirely changed my perception of my body. I learned how my thoughts and feelings influenced my biochemistry, and it entirely changed the way I was approaching my mental and psycho-emotional life.

I learned about functional medicine, and it entirely changed my views on the conventional medical and health-care system. I learned about how our collective, epidemic health challenges are both reflecting and worsening our world's biggest social, economic, and environmental problems, and it entirely changed my thinking about what health really means.

Learning all of this radicalized me. In many ways, it inspired and motivated me at a deep level. In other ways, it made me angry and outraged. I felt oppressed and like the world was a really unfair, messed-up place. I began channeling my frustration against the Unhealthy Default Reality, rather than toward myself. In the process, I did a lot of waving my fist in the air, a lot of ranting and railing about greed, corruption, and injustice.

That was gratifying at first. But after a while it got old. It got tiring. I decided it wasn't enough to be aware of the problems and outraged about them. I wanted to be part of the solution.

Slowly but surely, over time, I began finding new ways of relating to the unhealthy world around me. Ways that allowed me to embrace my inner rebel without allowing her to run my life, or run me ragged.

I decided that the best thing I could do to make my own life healthier while also trying to make the world a healthier place was to keep on learning and sharing the best of what I discovered actually worked. So, for the past fifteen years or so, that's pretty much what I've been doing.

Your story: To what extent have you gotten serious about owning your health, stewarding it, and safeguarding it as an expression of your individual life force? Have you resisted being defined by a diagnosis, disease state, or other pathological label? Have you come to question conventional, superficially defined ideals of health and fitness? To what extent have you become willing to experiment, build skills, and explore alternative solutions to your own health-and-happiness challenges? What energizes and entices you now? What depletes or disempowers you?

Areas for review: The value of becoming your own rescuer. Safeguarding your sanity; building your capacity and skills. Embracing a damn-the-torpedoes mindset. Dealing with doubt, criticism, disapproval, resistance, ridicule, and jealousy. Surrendering your attachment to being good enough, right, perfect, or even normal. Working within your available means and known strengths. Discerning between real and fake role models.

Reflect for a moment on these areas of inquiry, and if you like, note your answers in a journal.

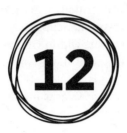

Act 7: Healthy Deviance

Ideas at first considered outrageous or ridiculous
or extreme gradually become what people
think they've always believed. How the transformation
happened is rarely remembered....
Our hope is in the dark around the edges,
not the limelight of center stage.
Our hope and often our power.

—REBECCA SOLNIT

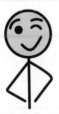

Figuring out how to live comfortably and sustainably as a healthy person in an unhealthy world was not something I learned overnight, or even over the course of a few years. It took realizing that I could not do it all. It took learning that I had to carefully bide my energy and time and not exhaust myself fighting too many "issues" at the expense of my own well-being. It took learning that my tendency is generally to take on way too much, and to value my own well-being way too little.

Over time, I made a lot of major changes. I moved from the major metro area where I'd been living back to the organic farm where I was raised. I got married, and then divorced, yet somehow managed to keep my ex as a good friend. I left *Experience Life* magazine for a coveted job at *Huffington Post* and then decided that job wasn't for me. I went back to *Experience Life* magazine, and then left again a couple years later, this time clear about how I could do that in peace and still keep doing what I loved. All the while, I tried different approaches to eating, to moving, to managing my life depending on the circumstances, my goals, and my desires. And always, I kept learning—what worked, what didn't, what I loved, and what left me feeling "meh." Each year was a little different than the year before.

I ultimately realized that I would need to practice health and happiness as a form of ongoing mastery—the way you might practice a sport or musical instrument or any skill that you are always looking to improve, and where your reasons for playing shift and become more nuanced over time.

Seeing my life this way—as an evolving journey rather than as some forced march in which I *must* comply with this or that diet or plan, in which I *must* achieve this or that bodily result—has been full of rewards. It has brought a much bigger, more beautiful picture into view. And sometimes I feel sad when I am reminded of how long it was *not* that way for me. I know that I still don't have all the answers, but I have come to appreciate the importance of asking the right questions. And I guess that's why I do what I've been doing, in one form or another, for close to two decades now. Through writing and editing, through speaking and teaching, through consulting, podcasting, and more.

Through all my study and experimentation, I've gotten clear on a few things, the most important of which is this:

It has to feel good.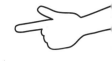

It might be challenging (like the week-long water fast I did a few years back). It might be weird (like the Three Walks exercise I present in chapter 18). It might even be maddening (like giving up my beloved tree nuts when they started putting holes in my tongue). But each of these things has also brought satisfaction and meaningful change. And beyond feeling good, that's the other thing I've found matters to me: *Meaning.*

The nice thing about doing something for decades is that you start to see evidence that at least some of it has made a difference. While to date, none of my work has resulted in wild riches or immense personal fame, it has produced a sense of satisfaction that I would not trade for the world (particularly since I have now met a lot of folks who have wild riches and immense personal fame, and I can tell you that it does not seem to have made most of them healthy or happy).

What's especially satisfying is observing that at least some my work has found its way around the world, and discovering that much of it seems surprisingly universal. For example, back in 2010, while working with Life Time Fitness and *Experience Life* magazine, I wrote a feature called "Being Healthy Is a Revolutionary Act: Perspectives for Thriving in a Mixed-Up World." As a removable insert for that feature, I penned a little chapbook, *A Manifesto for Thriving in a Mixed-Up World*. We even launched a companion website and a mobile app called "101 Revolutionary Ways to Be Healthy." Suddenly, I started hearing from people in far-flung places that this work was making a difference to them and that I was speaking a truth that other people recognized as their own.

In 2012, I met Queen Rania of Jordan at the Davos World Economic Forum (through Mark Hyman and Arianna Huffington—long story) and I learned that this actual queen (!) had been reading the magazine for years. She said she felt its messages were important ones for all people (and especially the women in her own culture) to hear.

Every once in a while, while traveling, I'll see the magazine in some unexpected place. I'll see a poster of the 101 Revolutionary Ways to Be Healthy up on a wall (I've heard U.S. Representative Tim Ryan has one in his congressional office). I'll see a quote from one of my columns in somebody else's blog. This is always kind of mind-blowing. It's a nice ego boost, sure, but more than that, it's a feeling of being part of something much, much bigger than me.

Last year, for example, I had the honor of delivering the opening keynote at the Ancestral Health Symposium in New Zealand, and while there, I got to hear from people all over the world who said this Healthy Deviant idea made sense to them. Many of them were sharing excitingly deviant ideas of their own—challenging assumptions and blind spots, pointing out flaws in the scientific evidence, offering experimental ways of approaching entrenched health challenges.

It's exciting to witness the gradual mainstreaming of Healthy Deviance, and the building of a progressive, intersecting health movement by all those who are intent on doing things differently. But even now, it's not always easy or intuitive. Often, it's bewildering, confounding, and downright tough.

With this in mind, a few years back I started a podcast with my friend Dallas Hartwig (of Whole30 fame). We called it *The Living Experiment,* reflecting on the fact that this way of being in the world does, in fact, require a huge amount of creative experimentation. The podcast title is also meant to reflect that those of us choosing to live this way are, in fact, living experiments of our own making. We are out here seeing what happens when we *don't* go along with the default program.

Most of us who are living this way acknowledge that we don't really have a formal map. We're traipsing and trudging along, exploring, reporting back from the field, and then exploring some more. This is the part of Healthy Deviance that I love the most—the experimenting and sharing, the learning and growing, the meeting other Healthy Deviants and discovering together how we can make our lives work, and at the same time, how we can get the world we all share to work better for everyone.

Somewhere in every Healthy Deviant Hero's Journey, I think the potential for this feeling exists—this feeling of clarity that it really does matter whether we are healthy and happy. Not because of how awesome we'll look, all of the fabulous things we will have, or how impressive we will appear to others. But because in being healthy and happy, we deliver more of the goods we are meant to deliver. We experience more of the goods we are meant to receive. And in this mysterious, rapidly unfolding universe of ours, where what comes around tends to go around, I believe that makes this world a kinder, gentler, more beautiful place for all of us to live.

Your story: To what extent can you identify a Healthy Deviant instinct within you? In what ways does the idea of forging your own Healthy Deviant identity appeal to you—and/or leave you cold? What natural strengths do you bring to your personal healthy-change efforts, and which, if any, do you feel inspired to share? How do you see the next chapters of your health journey going?

Areas for review: The value of moving from self-improvement to self-discovery and self-expression. The priority of sustainability over quick, superficial results. Finding your own healthy, right-now version of perfection. Getting comfortable in your own body-mind and releasing your negative judgments of it. Locating the Healthy Deviants in your midst, even when (at first) there don't seem to be any. Setting your own course and finding your next clear step.

Reflect for a moment on these areas of inquiry, and if you like, note your answers in a journal.

Are You a Healthy Deviant?
(Take the Quiz!)

By now you have probably figured out that this is not your average health book. Accordingly, I figure that the chances you are still reading this book and *not* some sort of Healthy Deviant are rather slim. But you can take my online "Are You a Healthy Deviant?" quiz to find out for sure—and to see where on the Healthy Deviant spectrum you currently fall. Just visit HealthyDeviant.com and hit the quiz button in the upper right corner. You'll answer twenty or so multiple-choice questions, and then—voila!—based on your score, you'll be placed into one of the following unscientific categories. (By the way, if you bristle at the idea of being placed into *any* predetermined category, you can give yourself an extra Healthy Deviant point for that. Go, you!)

TOTAL OF 0 TO 10: DECIDEDLY NON-DEVIANT

This score suggests that you prefer to take a more conventional approach to your health-related decisions. Alternatively, it could reflect that you are just starting out on your health journey or that your health isn't currently a top priority for you (perhaps because you have a lot of other pressing concerns at this time). Even so, you might benefit from learning more about Healthy Deviance as a way of understanding a health-motivated friend or loved one, expanding your own health-seeking horizons, or better understanding emerging health and wellness trends.

TOTAL OF 11 TO 60: HEALTHY DEVIANT IN THE MAKING

This score suggests that you are already well on your way to embracing a progressive, nonconformist approach to health improvement and healthy living. Whether or not you personally identify with the term *Healthy Deviant*, you share at least some attitudes and experiences common to Healthy Deviants, and you dabble with unconventional mindsets and solutions from time to time. You will probably enjoy learning more about

Healthy Deviance, and would benefit from continuing to develop your Healthy Deviant skills and strengths.

TOTAL OF 61 TO 80: HEALTHY DEVIANT

This score suggest that you possess many of the classic hallmarks of a nonconformist health seeker, and that you probably have already had a fair bit of experience navigating the confusing realms of health improvement. Whether or not you identify as a Healthy Deviant, you probably relate to a lot of the challenges faced by them. You might also have experienced some of the rewards of resisting the pull of our unhealthy culture (even when that's tough to do). If you're like most Healthy Deviants, you are on a path toward lifelong learning and experimentation in the service of your health and happiness. You likely find satisfaction in sharing what you know with others.

TOTAL OF 81 TO 100: HARDCORE HEALTHY DEVIANT

This score suggests that you take your health pretty darn seriously, and you're willing to stray well outside the bounds of so-called normalcy in order to live in harmony with your own healthy values and priorities. You are probably a bit of a renegade outlier—and you are okay with that. You may be disappointed or even dismayed at times by the unhealthy state of the world, but you are also a proactive change agent, intent on doing what you can to make it a healthier, happier place for yourself and others. You are already walking the path of the Healthy Deviant and always interested in discovering resources that will help support you on the next phases of that journey. It's likely that many people see you as a role model of healthy living. If you choose, inspiring others toward health and happiness could become an increasingly big part of your life.

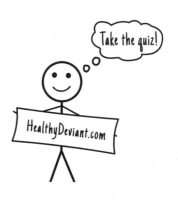

Take the quiz!

HealthyDeviant.com

From Suffering to Self-Authorship

No matter what your score on the "Are You a Healthy Deviant?" quiz, and regardless which of the above descriptions sounds more like you, please know that there is no right or wrong place to be on the Healthy Deviant spectrum. Every spot has unique purpose and value. Each has distinct lessons and gifts. You can become healthy from any position, if you choose.

The central goal of Healthy Deviance is not to create some special club where you are either in or out. It's to offer you some fun, alternative, and creative ways to go about being a healthy person in a predominantly unhealthy world, if you choose.

What matters is not that you decide to take on some externally recognized label. What matters is that as you redefine your relationship with the UDR, you forge an identity of your own making. Little by little, you cease living at the mercy of your circumstances, conforming with what is expected of you. You begin consciously authoring your own story, reclaiming your autonomy, and renegotiating your existence on your own terms.

When progress is no longer measured just by pounds on the scale, the size of your jeans, your adherence to a particular diet, or your ability to look like or impress some other person, the game is changed. And when you stop losing at the willpower-and-compliance-oriented game of self-improvement and start winning at the awareness-and-autonomy-oriented game of Healthy Deviance, life gets dramatically more interesting and rewarding. It becomes a flow experience of its own accord.

Right now, if you're stuck in the frustrating cycles of ego depletion and learned helplessness, that promise of flow may seem out of reach. Please know: *This is an illusion. It's a parlor trick of the UDR. Don't fall for it.*

In this game, you can change course, change views, and change positions at any time. Solutions are often much closer than they appear.

No matter where your experience within the UDR has taken you up till now, you can rewrite your own story's next chapter. And as you reassert your rights to that story, you will find that the UDR loses its claim on you.

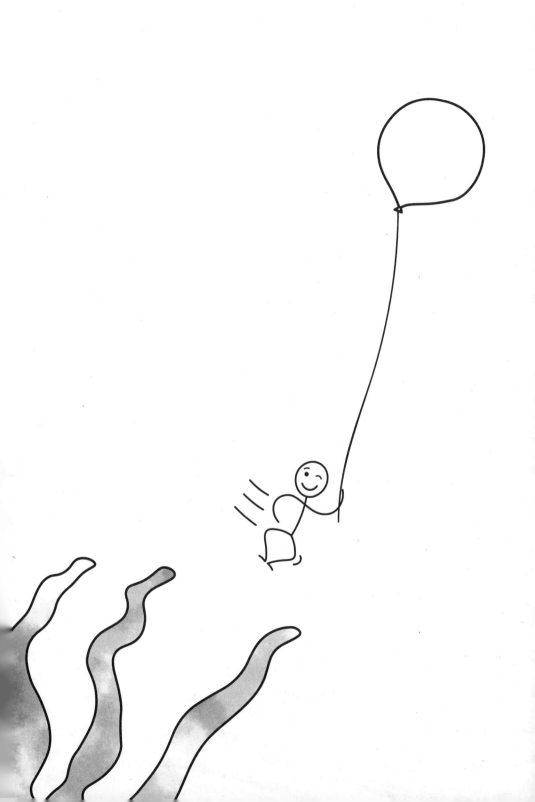

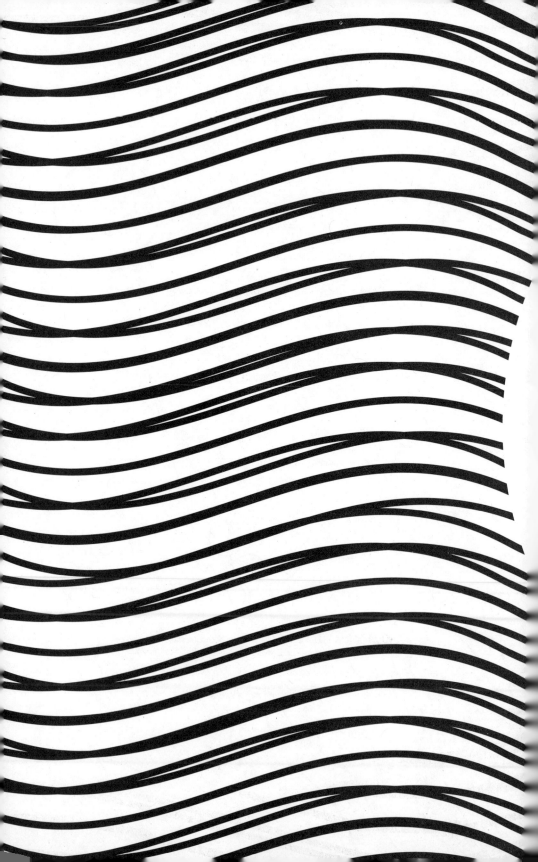

PART 3

The Way of the Healthy Deviant

"This is my way; where is yours?"—
Thus I answered those who asked me "the way."
For the way—that does not exist.

—FRIEDRICH NIETZSCHE, *THUS SPOKE ZARATHUSTRA*

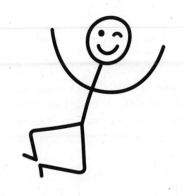

The Nonconformist Competencies

> To be yourself in a world that is
> constantly trying to make you something else
> is the greatest accomplishment.
>
> —RALPH WALDO EMERSON

By now, I'm hoping you are beginning to formulate a different, more honoring and dignified sense of your own health struggles. I'm hoping you are starting to see that healthy change eludes most of us *not* because we lack self-discipline, but rather because the Unhealthy Default Reality (UDR) in which we are all living disrupts our mechanisms of self-regulation.

Subsisting within the UDR exhausts our available resources. It saps our conscious awareness and autonomy. It erodes our confidence and self-regard. It results in chronic inflammatory damage and depletion that, unless countered, dramatically reduce our capacity to effect positive change. It makes us vulnerable to all manner of unhealthy temptations and self-numbing agents that drag us down even further.

Practicing the Nonconformist Competencies of Healthy Deviance helps you avoid that fate and empowers you to expand your Healthy Deviant mojo. There are a whole bundle of Nonconformist Competencies that most Healthy Deviants gradually develop and continue to master over time, but here are the three master competencies I see as mattering most:

- Amplified Awareness

- Preemptive Repair

- Continuous Growth and Learning

Read on to learn more about each of them and to get a sense of how you can put them to work in the service of your own well-being. Embracing them will help you wiggle free of the UDR's grip and get a much firmer grasp on what matters to you.

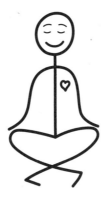

Amplified Awareness

A motivated observer develops faculties
that a casual spectator may never be aware of.

—EVELYN FOX KELLER

In a society that presents us with a ceaseless barrage of attention-gobbling distractions, temptations, demands, and unhealthy default choices, cultivating conscious awareness is an essential health-preserving defense. Because unless you're aware enough to notice your imperiling circumstances, much like the proverbial frog in hot water, you're not going to be inclined to change or challenge your situation until it's too late.

So the first requirement of Healthy Deviance is waking up to your reality, and then *staying* awake enough that you are able to track what is actually happening, both within and around you. The Healthy Deviant Adventure program presents a collection of proven strategies for doing just that while *also* building resilience in the face of forces that might currently be getting the better of you.

Starting first thing in the morning, when you wake up, at regular intervals throughout the day, and right up until the time you go to sleep, you'll learn to reclaim and progressively protect your own head space. In the process, you'll learn to spot the ways you're inclined to abdicate your awareness in favor of external stimulation, zoning out, or the comfort of "just going along" with the path of least resistance. (See the "Your Trouble Clock" exercise in chapter 19).

In effect, you'll learn to become more aware of the consequences of both the choices *and the non-choices* you're currently making, and to identify your highest-leverage opportunities for intervention. And once you've mastered the art of managing your own awareness, you'll witness how much easier and more rewarding healthier choices become. You'll be surprised by how much more quickly you're able to hop out of any hot water in which you happen to find yourself.

The reason I chose Amplified Awareness as the first Nonconformist Competency is that Healthy Deviance begins with noticing your relationship to a dominant culture—a culture that influences you in a thousand ways on a daily basis. Most people are simply not aware of that relationship and have never given those influences much thought. Without the awareness, there can be no real deviance. There can be no choice to differ from unhealthy norms in ways that benefit you. There can only be a reaction, an unconscious resistance and frustration and suffering. All of which depletes you. And inflames you. And makes you nuts.

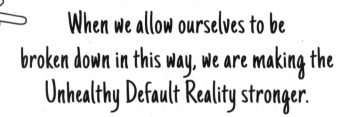

When we allow ourselves to be broken down in this way, we are making the Unhealthy Default Reality stronger.

Amplified Awareness is the first and most essential step in ceasing that pattern.

Amplified Awareness Basics

WHAT IT'S ABOUT
The ability to notice, accurately assess, and consciously respond to what is going on within and around you, including important signals you've probably been overlooking or actively ignoring for a long time.

WHY IT'S IMPORTANT
If you don't notice how and when the Unhealthy Default Reality is messing with you, you can't fight back. If you can't recognize the telltale signs that you are becoming worn down, worked up, inflamed, or overwhelmed, you stand no chance of avoiding next-level damage and disempowerment. With

awareness comes autonomy and conscious choice; without it, you become a perennial victim of circumstance.

Strategies for Building Amplified Awareness

- **Slow down:** Several times a day, especially when you're feeling stressed, purposefully slow your pace and deepen your breathing; assume a relaxed, upright, "here and now" posture; and notice your mind shifting into a similar gear.

- **Tune out and tap in:** As often as you can, turn off external noise from all electronics and mass media in favor of tracking your own thoughts, feelings, and impulses, as well as noticing what is going on around you.

- **Ask questions:** When you are feeling triggered, tempted, reactive, or depleted, or when you are suffering the aftermath of an unhealthy decision, ask: "What just happened? What current or recent factors led up to this? What are my choices in this moment?" Listen for your own wise answers.

Helpful Amplified Awareness Practices

Here are some simple practices that help build Amplified Awareness:

- Scheduled "nothing" time
- Non-rushing
- Deep breathing
- Mindfulness meditation
- Self-observation, reflection, journaling
- Coaching and therapy
- Yoga
- Conscious eating
- Conscious commuting
- Curious, non-directed gazing
- Active listening

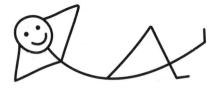

Preemptive Repair

We're in an era of great breakdown ...
and when systems break down,
the ones who have the resilience
to actually repair themselves,
they move to a higher order of organization.

—JOAN HALIFAX

We've seen how living in a culture rife with pressures, demands, and temptations plays out in our body-minds. We incur a lot of damage. Our systems get weakened. Our defenses get worn down. Our resilience gets compromised. Our sense of identity and purpose get warped. Then we get hit with that self-perpetuating vicious cycle of the Unhealthy Default Reality (UDR). *The less healthy and fit we are, the harder it is to do the things that would improve our health and fitness.*

This is not just a mental game. Excess abdominal fat drives unhealthy cravings and undermines metabolism. A lack of fitness saps your energy, strength, and desire to move. A lack of sleep undermines your hormones and neurotransmitters and prevents your body from repairing and detoxifying cell tissue. All of this leads to increased inflammation and lowered (or overactive) immunity throughout the body. Those conditions lead to chronic disease states that dramatically complicate and limit our lives—making it harder still to take health-improving steps. And, of course, all of that leads to reduced mental and emotional capacity, lowered mood, and so on.

Fortunately, there's a potential bright side here. We know that the growth of new muscle occurs when stressed, damaged muscle is repaired and, in the process, reinforced.

As you repeatedly encounter and repair the damage incurred by living in an unhealthy culture, you can get stronger.

As you apply Amplified Awareness, your instincts get better. Your perception is heightened. Your capacity expands. Your equanimity, resilience, and endurance improve. You can then transfer those newfound strengths, applying them in the service of your highest choices, desires, and acts of self-expression. Without adequate opportunity to repair, though, such gains are impossible. Instead, the damage accumulates and leaves you increasingly weakened and disempowered. Which is why you need strategies for regenerating your energy, hope, and resilience faster than the mass-culture machine can deplete them.

This is not about dragging ourselves to bed when we are no longer able to think straight or eating an "energy bar" when our blood sugar bottoms out. It's about knowing that we cannot let the UDR get its fangs into us that deeply before we take evasive action. Instead of emphasizing rest and recovery only *after* we've exhausted ourselves, we have to begin preemptively repairing and proactively rebalance ourselves at the cellular, biochemical, neurological, and psychological level.

The 14-Day Healthy Deviant Adventure program helps you instill just such Preemptive Repair practices, giving you the best possible advantage in maintaining your health and happiness for the long haul. And here's the great news: Reversing the direction of your trajectory—from self-weakening damage (downward spiral) to self-strengthening repair (upward spiral)—can start with a single, empowering choice.

The Renegade Rituals (especially Ultradian Rhythm Breaks) teach you how to better predict, notice, and respond to your own signals of physical, mental, emotional, and spiritual depletion. They teach you ways of relating to an often-hostile environment without becoming victimized by it. Rather than feeling continually at war with your circumstances, these strategies help you frame the dynamic tension as a challenging quest, a tango-like dance, an athletic challenge, or an advanced martial arts practice, one in which you develop exceptional strengths, talents, and capacities. One in which you get stronger as you go.

Preemptive Repair Basics

The willingness to regularly replenish, restore, and strategically reinforce depleted systems *before* they render you vulnerable, oblivious, incapacitated, or dangerously reactive.

We live in a culture that generates a near constant supply of inflammatory stressors and that massively undervalues rest and recovery. Just by virtue of existing on the midst of our society's unhealthy norms and overwhelming demands, our physical, mental, and emotional resilience are constantly being depleted.

Unless you prioritize Preemptive Repair strategies, your body's delicate tissues will get irritated. Your nervous system will get overloaded. Your biochemistry will get imbalanced. Your moods will become destabilized. Your healthy priorities and choices will be undermined. Your energy will be squandered and drained. To avoid that, you have to get ahead of the damage being done to you on a daily basis, resting before you are exhausted, replenishing your reserves before you get seriously ill, proactively repairing and rebuilding your body and mind while you still have the wherewithal to do so.

Strategies for Preemptive Repair

- **Run offense and defense:** Recognize that our culture generally won't prompt you to rest, take breaks, or prioritize self-repair until after you've broken down. Accept that you'll have to actively elbow out space and time for your Preemptive Repair priorities, while also maintaining strong boundaries to defend them.

- **Play the long game:** Taking a few minutes or hours to rest and recover early can save you days or weeks you could otherwise lose to sickness, injury, accidents, mistakes, or missed opportunities. Every hour you spend in a high-vitality state is an hour with a much higher likelihood of big ideas, satisfying experiences, and other great payoffs.

- **Get into agreement with your body:** It generally doesn't tell you to rest unless it needs to rest. If it's asking for a break, that's because said break is in your best interest. It's also quite possibly the only thing standing between you and some life crisis with a high price tag. Start by listening to the small signals. When your body tells you it wants a glass of water, a hug, a walk around the block, a few minutes of sunshine, an extra hour of sleep, or to go pee, make that happen, ASAP.

Smart Preemptive Repair Practices

Here are some simple practices that help you embrace Preemptive Repair:

- Sleep, rest, relaxation
- Recovery days
- Ultradian Rhythm Breaks (see Renegade Rituals, below)
- Mindfulness practices and meditation
- Peace and quiet
- Good nutrition and hydration
- Detoxification
- Deep breathing
- Moderate activity
- Bodywork
- Creative outlets
- Time in nature
- Self-care
- Laughter
- Time spent with loved ones
- Healthy sensual activity
- Good integrative health-care support

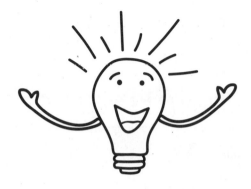

Continuous Growth and Learning

Once you stop learning, you start dying.

—ALBERT EINSTEIN

Just as living in a forest, jungle, desert, or other wilderness setting requires a set of specialized survival skills and sensibilities, so does the challenge of thriving in our supposedly "civilized" modern environments. To thrive in an unhealthy culture, you need to master skills for nourishing and defending not just your body but also your mind, heart, and spirit. You need strategies for locating healthy options in a sea of unhealthy default choices, for avoiding common traps and obstacles, and for minimizing collateral damage.

Beyond the basic block-and-tackle of nutrition, exercise, and sleep, these lesser-appreciated skills include things like mindset and mood adjustment, time and energy management, media literacy, self-directed health-care savvy, and more. These are skill sets that most sustainably healthy people know and practice, and that most chronically unhealthy people have not learned to consistently embrace—yet.

These are the survival skills of the new era.

But here's the deal. You cannot possibly learn all these skills all at once. You can no more hope to instantly master them all any more than you can wander into the woods and hope to master wilderness survival in a day. So it's important to acquire the most basic skills first and then embark on a life-long, intrinsically rewarding pursuit of the more advanced and subtle ones.

Right, so what are the most essential skills—the one it helps to build *first*? In my view, they are the first two Nonconformist Competencies, Amplified Awareness and Preemptive Repair (which is, of course, why I started with them). And then we get into this third Nonconformist Competency, Continuous Growth and Learning. This means, quite literally, learning how to learn. For starters, you have to get comfortable with the fact that you do not already know it all and that you cannot possibly learn everything you need to know by looking to celebrity role models and quick-tip listicles for all your answers.

Getting Your Priorities Straight

In wilderness survival, they emphasize doing things in a particular order that will help you not panic and not die before help arrives. Most survival manuals suggest you first find or make a shelter (to avoid exposure, the factor that kills most quickly). *Then* you can work on finding water. *Then* on making a fire. Only after you've done those things should you begin worrying about food.

In Healthy Deviant survival, I think it helps to follow a similar set of priorities. Amplified Awareness, Preemptive Repair, and Continuous Growth and Learning are, in my mind, the shelter-water-fire priorities of a healthy life. From there, we'll get to all that other diet-and-exercise stuff as a matter of course.

The truth is, you don't really need to know how many calories and what precise combination of macronutrients to eat on Monday, Wednesday, and Friday. You don't necessarily need to know how to do sets and reps and sprints and intervals and heart-rate training. You don't need to precisely measure your ketones or track every step you take. Certainly, amassing and tracking that kind of information can be fun and motivating for some people. But for some it can be overwhelming, distracting, an exercise in futility. And one of the biggest problems with focusing on all the "must-know" minutia we're pressured to learn is that it completely distracts and discourages us from learning the skills that matter more.

Here are the key, survival-level quandaries most of us are facing right now:

- How do I notice what's going on within and around me and stay true to my own priorities when distractions and temptations are everywhere?

- How can I remain sane and nonreactive in the midst of total madness?

- How do I find the time, energy, focus, skill, and resources to make healthy choices in a world that makes them much harder than unhealthy ones?

Almost invariably, though, people in our culture are encouraged to just start with diet and exercise. They think *they have to* start with diet and exercise. And yet they are totally befuddled and overwhelmed by diet and exercise. "Just tell me what to eat!" they beg. "Just tell me what to do!"

I've been there. I can relate. And look, if that's *really* what you want, I've provided a long list of suggestions in chapter 18, "Healthy Deviant Survival Skills," to get you started. I suspect, however, that if you could easily do most of the things I've listed there, you'd probably have done them already. Maybe you have, and maybe you haven't. And if you haven't or feel you can't, please know that this does not reflect some inherent weakness or failure on your part.

Learning to eat and enjoy whole foods, as I've noted, is one of the most powerful changes you can make for your health, sanity, and well-being. Once you are eating well, you'll have much better energy and mental clarity and feel more capable of doing all sorts of other things that are great for you, like moving and challenging your body to get stronger. You'll sleep better. Your mood will improve. So, *if* your food is something you feel you can have solid success in changing, and *if* you can manage to do that in your current body-mind state, then yeah, food is a great place to start.

But eating mostly whole foods involves a whole *slew* of skills: Not just knowing what whole foods are but also knowing how to find them in environments where they are often scarce; knowing how to choose, store, prepare, and combine them so they taste great and feel satisfying; knowing which ones agree with you and which ones don't; knowing how to integrate them into your busy, life; and knowing how to prioritize them even when you are being actively incentivized and encouraged to eat all sorts of other processed crap.

My friend and podcasting partner Dallas Hartwig has coauthored two terrific *New York Times*–bestselling books, *It Starts with Food* and *The Whole 30*. I want to say, straight up, that if you are feeling deeply inspired to "start with food," both would be great books to read and begin adjusting your eating around. For a lot of people, though (and maybe you are one of them?), food is so charged with shame and misery and regret and trouble—and they feel so out of control around their food—that food is *not at all* the best place to start. Certainly, that was true of me for a long time.

Ultimately, you can decide for yourself which healthy skills you want to focus on first. Just keep in mind that in embracing Healthy Deviance, you will need to learn how to steward not just your body but also your mind, your relationships, your environment, and your way of being in the world. If you judge yourself harshly for "not knowing how," if you give in to hopelessness and despair because being healthy is "too hard," you are playing into the system that is breaking you down. Remember:

We're not doing that here.

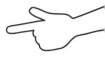

Continuous Growth and Learning Basics

WHAT IT'S ABOUT
The enthusiastic, ongoing expansion your healthy-person skill set using a "growth mindset"[30]—one that assumes you are capable of learning anything you need to know and that greets each new challenge as an opportunity to grow.

WHY IT'S IMPORTANT
The main thing separating most healthy people from most unhealthy people is that the healthy people have mastered a bunch of skills that the unhealthy folks haven't—yet. These aren't just skills related to diet and exercise, as noted, but also skills related to stress, sleep, media, medicine, consumer savvy, community building, mindfulness, and so much more.

Strategies for Continuous Growth and Learning

- **Be patient and persistent, and when you need to be, be plodding:** Start with basics (like the Renegade Rituals) and enthusiastically embrace the fact that you will always be learning and growing, because the world will continue to change, and so will you.

- **Take a "beginner's mind" approach:** If you judge yourself harshly for "not knowing how," if you give into frustration and despair because being healthy is "too hard," or because you're "not good enough," you are playing right into the system that is messing with your mojo. Stop doing that! Instead, simply decide that you can and will learn whatever you need to learn to be healthy, and then start where you are—now.

- **Celebrate progress and small successes:** Successful growth requires curiosity, practice, and experimentation. It also requires noticing and celebrating even the smallest bits of incremental progress. You figured out a new way to pack a healthy lunch? Yay! You cut back a bit on your nighttime television watching? Woo hoo! You handled a recurrent conflict with your partner in a way that worked slightly better than last time? You win! Every step in the direction of your well-being is a good step.

Continuous Growth and Learning Practices

Here are some simple practices that help your pursue Continuous Growth and Learning:

- Reading books, magazines, blogs, newspapers, and scientific journals
- Taking courses, seminars, and workshops
- Watching videos and documentary films
- Listening to podcasts, radio shows, or books on tape
- Consulting with wise teachers and coaches
- Surrounding yourself with healthy friends and peers
- Systematic experimentation
- Assuming attitudes of curiosity, inquiry, and "beginner's mind"

Note: Some learning resources are great. Some are mind-numbing or misleading. To separate the good from the garbage, you'll need the skills of discernment and BS-detection. Amplified Awareness helps with that!

In closing this chapter on the Nonconformist Competencies, I want to leave you with one parting thought:

If you want to be a healthy person in an unhealthy culture, you're choosing the less-chosen path.

Things won't be arranged for you. You will be arranging them for yourself. You'll be figuring out how to do things most people never do. So why not start now—with the Renegade Rituals?

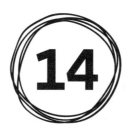

The Renegade Rituals

A ritual is the enactment of a myth. And, by participating in
the ritual, you are participating in the myth…. Your consciousness
is being re-minded of the wisdom of your own life.

—JOSEPH CAMPBELL

The Renegade Rituals serve many purposes. They are daily reminders and affirmations (to yourself and others) that you matter, that your well-being matters, that your life matters. They are your all-access pass to feeling better and thinking more clearly than most people do most of the time. Finally, they are your get-out-of-jail-free cards, always good for busting loose from the Unhealthy Default Reality's grip.

The Nobel Prize–winning poet Derek Walcott once said, "Any serious attempt to try to do something worthwhile is ritualistic." And I could not agree more. These rituals, like most rituals, return to you what you put into them. They don't have to be fancy or complicated. They just need to be taken as matters of importance. Eminently worthwhile in their own right, they become even more so if you regard them as semi-sacred and regularly allocate even a small amount of your time and attention to performing them with consistency and care.

The Renegade Rituals include:

- **The Morning Minutes:** A brief, pleasant morning ritual designed to help you reclaim your waking moments and better manage whatever the world throws your way.

- **Ultradian Rhythm Breaks (URBs):** Short, periodic rest periods that optimize your capacity by supporting your body's natural energy cycles, self-regulation mechanisms, and critical repair processes.

- **The Nighttime Wind-Down Ritual:** A calming pre-sleep transition for your body and mind, designed to help you get much-needed rest, marshal essential resources, and create the conditions for next-day resilience and success.

Taken together, these simple practices form the structural backbone of the Healthy Deviant Adventure program. They also help you develop the figurative "backbone" required to stay your chosen course, and defend yourself against unhealthy influences. Repeated regularly, these practices provide the foundation for healthy autonomy while maximizing vitality and productivity. They also make your life more pleasurable and rewarding—providing whole-person nourishment, recovery, and relief that you've probably been missing.

But perhaps the most valuable thing about these rituals is their ability to help you perceive clearly what is *really* getting in the way of you being healthy. When you struggle to do these practices, when you're tempted to skip them, when you "forget" to do them, or when you are blocked from doing them, notice with keen interest:

Why does that happen?
How does that happen?

I'm going to describe the details of each Renegade Ritual in separate chapters, but before I do, I want to give you a better understanding of their framework, and the reason I've included them here (rather than, say, a particular set of diet or exercise strategies).

The Dynamics of Doing and Not Doing

There's a Zen saying: *How you do anything is how you do everything.*

Guess what? That includes how you go about *not* doing (i.e., avoiding, procrastinating, or "failing" to do) all the things you've committed to doing or been longing to do, but haven't.

In other words, how you *don't* do a given thing to support your own health and well-being is probably also how you go about *not doing a whole bunch of other things* that support your health and well-being. So, it's worth noticing: What gets in the way of your embracing these simple, pleasurable, self-sustaining daily practices?

Go ahead and make a list of what you predict could make them challenging, or what you know has made them challenging in the past. Lack of time and energy? Warring priorities? Other people? Media distractions? The lure of established patterns? The intrusion of unanticipated temptations? Go ahead—write 'em down, starting with your top five likely barriers:

1. _____

2. _____

3. _____

4. _____

5. _____

Whatever the reasons, whatever the barriers, please note that they are likely the same reasons and barriers that are getting in the way of a whole lot of *other* self-sustaining choices (like eating healthy, getting exercise) that you either want to do or think you "should" do.

Since the Renegade Rituals don't involve diet and exercise, though, and since they don't require much time or effort or any special skills, energy, resources, or preparation, the barriers to doing them are both lower and much easier to see for what they are: *Not* some fatal lack of willpower on your part, but culturally imposed, socially institutionalized blockades that are programmed into our so-called normal way of living. Becoming aware of the obstacles implicit in that way of living—actively studying them and their persistence in the Unhealthy Default Reality, and then learning to work around them—has an astonishing effect: It empowers you to relate differently and more successfully to *all* the obstacles within the Unhealthy Default Reality.

Moving into Micro-Action

The Healthy Deviant Adventure program gives you the opportunity to experiment with incorporating one or more Renegade Rituals into your days. You don't have to do them all. To start with, you might try one or two. Shrink them down, if you need to. Simplify them. Perform one bit or aspect of them for as little as one minute. Make the effort so negligible and so simple so you can't reasonably tell yourself that you "don't have time" or that it's "too hard."

If even a tiny effort feels like too much, just ask yourself, "What do I think would happen if I *did* try this, for just one minute, right now?" Do you feel a little burst of hope or energy? A spurt of emotion? A little breeze of clarity or possibility? That's good! Keep going with that! Then *find out* what would happen!

Do one micro-version of any of the Renegade Rituals described in the following chapters. Consider it an experiment. See what happens. Build in more of the Renegade Rituals as you feel ready. Greater regularity and frequency generally delivers better results, but the important thing is to start where you are, right now, and just do what you can.

If you proceed with an attitude of curiosity and willingness—willingness to defy the norms of the Unhealthy Default Reality and to wiggle loose of its grip on you, even just a little—you will gradually reclaim your ownership and authorship of yourself. That, my friends, is what Healthy Deviance is all about.

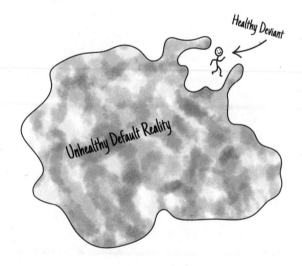

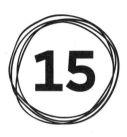

15

Morning Minutes

Caring for myself is not self-indulgence. It is self-preservation.
And that is an act of political warfare.

—AUDRE LORDE

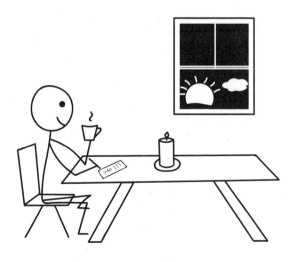

Do you know how most Americans wake up? They jolt awake to an alarm, flip on bright lights, reach for their electronic devices, then dive directly into their day's activities and responsibilities. They check email and texts, scan social feeds and news headlines to see what they might have missed while they slept. Seconds after their feet hit the floor, they switch on the television or radio to hear the familiar prattle of morning-show hosts or the dire pronouncements of news anchors; they turn on loud, hyper-intense music or hop on treadmills to get their blood pumping. Others jump into productive tasks, returning emails and calls, responding to requests for information, finishing up last-minute assignments before they have to go to work.

Typically, before most U.S. adults have had their first cup of coffee, their bodies are already in a state of high alert. Their bloodstreams are awash in an inflammatory cascade of cortisol and adrenaline. Their brains are flooded with new information, buzzing with new things to think, do, and react to.

As a Healthy Deviant, you're going to do your morning a bit differently. For your sanity, for your health, and for the benefit of everything you hold dear, you are going to consciously reclaim the first few moments of your day—for you. Rather than abruptly throwing some big industrial on-off lever into the "ON" position, you're going to turn your delicate dials at a pace your body and brain can handle. And for that, you will be richly rewarded, because from here on out, every single part of your day is going to go better.

The Morning Minutes practice is a simple, three-minute, day-starting routine that will help you stand strong in the face of whatever challenges, stresses, temptations, and consciousness-shutdowns the mass-culture machine has to throw at you today. If you are going to initially dabble with just one Renegade Ritual, I would start with this one, because it will give you an immediate sense of how one simple act of Healthy Deviance can create a wedge between you and the unconscious, automatic habits that hold most in their sway.

Waking more gently lets you take advantage of the important theta-brain-wave state and ramp up more gradually toward demanding tasks. Regularly adhering to a Morning Minutes practice also helps you build self-efficacy, develop mindfulness and equanimity, and start the day on your own terms. So let's do this thing!

Morning Minutes Basics

HOW?

- First thing on rising, before you do anything else (especially looking at your phone), choose any low-key, feel-good activity and just enjoy it for at least three minutes, or for as long as you find rewarding and doable (see more step-by-step tips on the next page).

- Before and during your Morning Minutes practice, avoid all exposure to electronics, media, and other sensory distractions or stressors. No email, texts, social media, or news until your body and mind have had a chance to come gradually and peacefully into their relaxed waking state.

- Some good Morning Minutes practice options include meditation, yoga, stretching, reading poetry or wisdom literature, journaling, or playing a musical instrument (see list below for more options).

- Consider using the last few moments of your practice to set your intentions for the day and visualize how you want it to go or to reflect on the things you are most grateful for.

WHY?

- Preserve and take advantage of the valuable "twilight" theta-brainwave state that exists between waking and sleeping—a highly suggestible state associated with insight, creativity, healing, lucidity, and deep awareness.

- Reduce the alarm response of the sympathetic nervous system and associated inflammatory cortisol spike.

- Spare your mind from exposure to stressful, distracting inputs and outside agendas when it is at its most impressionable.

- Build your capacity for self-regulation and your sense of self-efficacy (the belief that you can do what you set out to do).

- Start your day on your own terms (rather than in reaction to outside forces).

- Build your "savoring" muscles—helping you develop the neurocircuitry for experiencing and registering positive, pleasurable experiences and harvesting the downstream dopamine rewards (see research by Eric Garland, PhD, on how savoring works to counter unhealthy addictive tendencies).[31]

- Establish an early state of mindfulness and equanimity, making it easier to retain and reclaim that state later in the day (during your Ultradian Rhythm Breaks, for example).

- Claim an early window of opportunity to establish your autonomy and identity as a Healthy Deviant and to carry that sense of sovereignty with you as go out to face the Unhealthy Default Reality.

- Notice barriers and attitudes that may be undoing other healthy intentions.

STEP-BY-STEP PRACTICE TIPS

- Wake to a pleasant, non-jarring signal or sound, ideally from something that is *not* your smartphone. I prefer Now & Zen's progressive-chime based alarm clocks and light-based, sunrise-mimicking alarm clocks (like Philips Wake-Up Light, Lumie Bodyclock Active Wake-Up Light, and MOSCHE Sunrise Alarm Clock), most of which also have audible-alarm backups), but low-key, wake-to-music options can work, too—just be sure you can easily turn off, turn over, cover up, or otherwise block any light-emitting displays.

- Keeping houselights low, if possible, go directly to your practice area. If you're a person who loves coffee, hot tea, or water first thing, feel free to make your preferred morning beverage to enjoy during your practice.

- Avoid all interaction with complex electronics, digital devices, media (including radio, television, and newspapers)—and ideally, any complex interactions with other people—until your Morning Minutes practice is complete.

- Light a candle (unscented, natural beeswax is my far-and-away favorite).

- Set a timer for a minimum of three minutes, take a breath, and settle yourself.

- Choose any feel-good activity (see list of suggestions below) and enjoy it for the period of time you have chosen, or for as long as desirable or doable.

- Close your practice with three deep, energizing breaths. While slowly inhaling and exhaling, consider creating a brief "snapshot" visualization or holding an intention for how you want your day to go.

- Blow out your candle. Then move on to the active part of your day, noticing how the three minutes you just invested in your own well-being changes your outlook and energy.

- Notice how you did (or did not do) the practice ("how you do everything is how you do everything").

- Track immediate and longer-term effects.

OPTIONAL MORNING MINUTES ACTIVITIES

What you do during your Morning Minutes window is entirely up to you. What's important is that you do it for a minimum of three blissful minutes.

- Look into the candle and zone out.

- Waft some essential oils around and breathe deeply.

- Pick and read a wisdom card or a short passage in a wisdom book.

- Meditate, pray, or do breathing exercises.

- Step outside to see the sunrise or watch the clouds go by.

- Listen to birds or the rustle of wind through an open window.

- Do yoga, stretch, foam-roller, or massage your hands and feet.

- Pet your dog or cat.

- Play a musical instrument.

- Doodle in sketchbook.

- Write a little poem or pen a love note to yourself or someone else.

- Envision one thing you'd like to see happen.

- Think about three things you're grateful for, taking one deep breath for each.

- If you are doing (or dabbling with) the Healthy Deviant Adventure program, review today's passage, peruse your Daily Deviance Journal Pages from recent days, or catch up with your Healthy Deviant Adventure Tracker.

- Just sit there, do nothing, and notice how that feels.

Remember, your minimum commitment for this practice is three minutes. You can go longer if you like (hey, if you can carve out the time, take a half hour or more!), but let three minutes be your base plan. Even at three minutes, you might be tempted to skip this apparently self-indulgent and unproductive practice. After all, you've got things to do! You are busy and important! People are relying on you!

All the more reason why this three minutes matters so mightily. How much will everyone in your world benefit from a saner and stronger you? Plenty. Keep in mind that *this* is how you reclaim your power to choose.

This is how your train your system to do something beyond the habitual and out of the ordinary.

You're going to be doing a lot of that down the road. But the path starts right here with this small, seemingly innocuous yet revolutionary act. This is your moment.

So enjoy. For three. Whole. Minutes.

When you are done with your practice, blow out your candle. Take one more deep breath as you watch the smoke waft gently upward. When you feel complete with the experience, mark it off on your Daily Deviance Journal Page.

Smell This

 I am a big fan of plant-based aromatherapy for reasons both scientific and sensory, so I encourage you to consider using this powerful body-mind tool as an adjunct to all your Renegade Rituals.

Our olfactory sense evokes instantaneous responses in the limbic centers of our brains, prompting quick, measurable shifts in mood and mental state. If you're interested in the science, there's plenty to review.[32] But even if you're skeptical, I would invite you to give aromatherapy with organic, plant based oils, essences, or infusions a try.

I have used most major brands of oils and flower essences at various times, and have enjoyed them all. I have, for many years, used and loved Katie Hess's Lotus Wei products. And I have recently also fallen in love with Jenny Pao's Nectar Essences "Breathe Me" blends. I like beginning my Morning Practice with her "Energy-Mood Boost" blend (citrusy). I often start my Ultradian Rhythm Breaks with her "Focus Brain Boost" blend (spearminty), and my Nighttime Wind-Down Ritual with her "Sleep" blend (lavendery).

Reflection: Did you do your Morning Minutes practice? Yes? Great! How did it feel? Did you not do it? Hmmm, interesting ... notice why. Write down the reason (or reasons).

_____

_____

_____

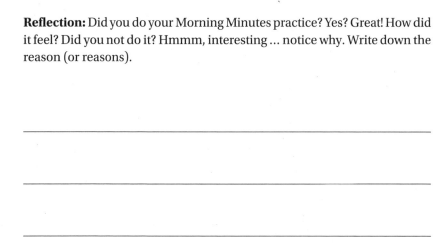

Both Lotus Wei and Nectar Essences integrate vibrational healing strategies and combine flower essences with essential oils, something that I find elevates these remedies over many other essential oil and aromatherapy products. But you can use whatever products you enjoy in any way you like. For the purposes of my Renegade Rituals, I tap just a drop or two out of an oil or essence blend on one palm, rub my hands together to release the aroma, then cup them in front of my face and inhale deep and slow. Ahhh.

My whole body-mind responds with an immediate focusing, enlivening, or settling response, depending on what I'm after. The combined experience is one of amplified pleasure (a great savoring practice). And with repeated use and association, I've found the aromas alone become powerful triggers for the ritual-ized responses I've trained my body-mind to expect. I can use that to my advantage for a quick sniff before a stressful meeting or as an alternative to an extra cup of mid-work session coffee.

If you don't have access to good essential oils, experiment with scratching the skin of a lemon or orange, cutting open a cucumber, or crushing a mint tea bag and smelling that instead.

Steal This Practice!

I developed my Morning Minutes ritual by co-opting (and then customizing) an idea from my younger sister, Andrea, a yoga teacher. Many years ago, having recently gotten her five-hundred-hour yoga-instructor certification from Kripalu, she had committed herself to doing thirty minutes of yoga each morning. It was an ambitious goal, so within a week or two, she found she was struggling (and often failing) to make that commitment work in the context of her daily life.

So instead of continuing to struggle or simply giving up, she radically re-designed the scope of her commitment. Her new plan was to simply unroll her mat, light some incense, kneel, and calmly taking three deep breaths. From there, she had the option of doing as much or as little yoga as she chose.

Of course, once she got to her mat, smelled the incense, settled in, and took her first breath, she often felt like stretching into a few asanas. From there, she might feel inspired to spend significantly more time on the mat, sometimes exceeding her original thirty-minute goal.

Envying both the beautiful experience my sister was giving herself, and the results she was getting, I tried copying her technique for a while. Over time, though, I realized that on some mornings, I didn't really want to do yoga. I was called to journal or meditate or play my guitar instead.

For me, the central appeal and core value of the practice lay in simply taking the first few minutes of the day for myself. So I expanded the range of potential practice activities to include anything calm, peaceful, and plea-surable that happened to appeal to me on that particular day.

I decided my minimum daily commitment would be three minutes, and I've been doing it ever since—sometimes for an hour or longer. On the rare days when I miss my Morning Minutes practice, I feel the difference, and I'm inspired to return to it, pronto. So, don't be shy about improvising with your own three-minute ritual—and creating your own versions of any of suggested exercises or practices in this book.

Remember—the goal is not for you to comply with any one set of steps or parameters that I prescribe; it's for you to establish healthy patterns you can enjoy for a lifetime. This simple, quiet, three-minute space is where all of your new patterns take root. Before the demands of the day and the Unhealthy Default Reality get the better of you.

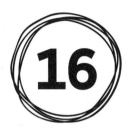

Ultradian Rhythm Breaks

Stress is basically a disconnection from the earth,
a forgetting of the breath. Stress is an ignorant state.
It believes that everything is an emergency.
Nothing is that important. Just lie down.

—NATALIE GOLDBERG

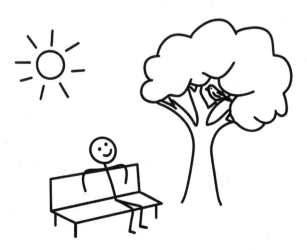

Never heard of ultradian rhythms? You are not alone. In all my health seeking and nearly two decades as a health journalist, I have only met a handful of people who were familiar with them, and they were mostly science nerds. But I want *you* to know about ultradian rhythms, because I am convinced that noticing and managing them well ranks in the top five most important (and marvelously deviant) things you can do for your well-being.

Although Ultradian Rhythm Breaks (which I call URBs for short) effectively serve and build all three Nonconformist Competencies (Amplified Awareness, Preemptive Repair, Continuous Growth and Learning), they are an especially perfect example of Preemptive Repair. They help your body and mind protect and rebuild themselves in the face of all sorts of daily assaults and stressors, they optimize your mental and physical performance, and they dramatically build your resilience to the Unhealthy Default Reality. That's why I consider Ultradian Rhythm Breaks an essential healthy-person skill, and why I have built them into the core of the 14-Day Healthy Deviant Adventure program.

Whole books (notably Ernest Rossi's *The 20-Minute Break*) and a great many scientific research papers have been written on the topic of ultradian rhythms, so if you're interested, I encourage you to read more about them. Here, I'm just going to tell you what you really need to know in order to become more aware of how ultradian rhythms operate in your daily life, and to make the most of the daily URBs that are central to your 14-Day Healthy Deviant Adventure experience.

The first thing to know is that ultradian rhythms are not some esoteric concept like chakras or third eyes (although I respect those things on their own merits). Rather, they are biological patterns hardwired into your DNA—a function of your "clock genes," which dictate how your body functions in time. Much like cardiac rhythms and brain waves, ultradian rhythms are measurable, observable, quantifiable physiological patterns that your body must maintain in order to operate properly.

Ultradian means "many times a day." *Rhythms* refers to the regular oscillating (up-and-down) wave patterns these cycles follow. The primary purpose of ultradian rhythms is to manage the cycles of energy production, output, and recovery that occur in all humans (as well as animals, plants, yeast, and fungi). Basically, ultradian rhythms are like mini-versions of circadian rhythms (our twenty-four-hour cycles of sleep and waking), except that they are much shorter, occurring many times over a single day. Like circadian rhythms, they have a powerful effect on your body, and when they are disrupted or ignored, they can really mess with your health, happiness, and general well-being. On paper, they look like this:

Ultradian Performance Rhythm

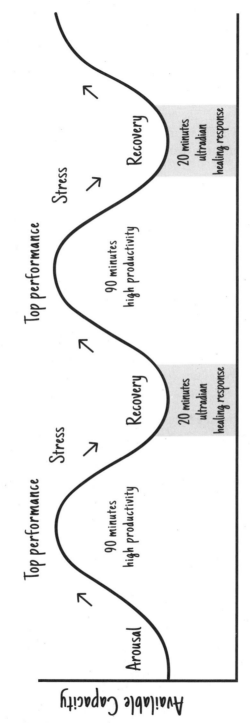

Course of Day

Illustration adapted from *The 20-Minute Break* by Ernest L. Rossi, PhD (Tarcher Putnam, 1991)

Your ultradian rhythms operate continually, day and night. While you're sleeping, they mostly affect things like your REM patterns, so you don't notice them much. During the day, however, they have a far more tangible impact on how you feel. Here's how your ultradian rhythms play out while you're going about your daily business:

- As you start your day and get yourself into a flow of sustained activity and mental focus, your body and brain start burning through a significant amount of oxygen, glucose, and other energetic fuels.

- Within about an hour and a half, you reach the apex of your productivity, entering what's known as an "ultradian performance peak."

- Meanwhile, the byproducts of all your mental and physical activity— metabolic waste, snippets of data, cellular debris—are building up in your system.

- After about an hour and a half or two hours, you begin experiencing this accumulation of all this detritus as stress. Your productivity and performance start to decline as your body enters what's known as an "ultradian trough"—an energetic low point.

- You start feeling fatigued, spacey, groggy, irritable, distracted, hungry, or fidgety. Your attention might wander. Your body might feel heavy, your face slack, your eyes glazed, unfocused, or droopy.

- You might feel the urge to hit the restroom, or you might experience a sudden craving for sugar, carbs, caffeine, or (if you smoke) a cigarette.

- You might also hear an anxious little internal voice saying, "Oh dear, it's only mid-morning and I'm already losing it. How am I going to make it through the day?"

Okay, freeze frame here: This is a super important moment— a moment of truth.

This is a moment to which you want to bring your newly amplified Healthy Deviant awareness. Because the feelings you're noticing right now? Those sloggy, tired, tweaky, distracted, "blah," or "ugh" feelings? These are signs that your body is working exactly as it should be. These are your body's flag-waving signals that it needs some down time—*now, or as soon as humanly possible*—in order to regenerate cellular fuel, rebalance your blood sugar and biochemistry, flush its detoxification systems, and repair damaged tissue.

Your brain also needs a break to sift through all the vast amounts of data you've taken in, tag it, organize it, and create important synaptic connections. These are the connections that allow your mental databases to merge and exchange information, producing those magical aha moments, creative insights, and brilliant solutions you kept wishing you had more of. These are the connections that allow important information currently piled up in your various mental inboxes to be sorted, labeled, and filed appropriately so that you can easily recall them later, whenever the need arises. These are the connections that determine whether you are a sparkling genius making great things happen or a grumpy, lumpen mass of flesh parked on an office chair wishing you were somewhere else.

In short, even if you don't care that much about your health and happiness, if you care at all about your brain and your career, these signals your body is sending you at this moment *matter*. So now, let's rejoin your body's ultradian program in action:

- Assuming you heed your body's signals for a break, the moment you step away from external demands and take a few deep breaths, your body's internal ground crews begin cranking into high gear, tackling a wide array of internal detoxification, maintenance, refueling, and repair tasks that comprise what's known as the "ultradian healing response."

- During the course of the next twenty minutes (ideally), fresh stores of fuel—in the form of adenosine triphosphate (ATP)—are delivered to your cells; blood sugar, hormones, and neurotransmitters are rebalanced; toxins are flushed; and many important fix-it and filing tasks are completed.

- At that point, your frontline systems ramp back up and rapidly return to full capacity for another hour and a half or two hours. Woo hoo!

But what if you ignore your body's signals and skip that break? Ah. I'm so glad you asked. Because frankly, that's exactly what most people choose to do. That's what I used to do, too, until I realized it was slowly killing me and undermining my ability to show up in my life.

Research shows (and my own experience confirms) that if we ignore our body's signals and white-knuckle our way through these low-energy dips, our energy and focus will eventually crawl out of the ultradian trough and return to a somewhat higher level of functioning—but not nearly as high as before. After a missed or skimped-on break, our next ultradian performance peak will be *significantly lower* than our previous one, which means we won't likely get as much done—or do it as well—and we also won't feel anywhere near as good while we are doing it. For the next hour and a half or two hours, our body and mind will keep slogging along, but at markedly reduced capacity.

If we miss subsequent breaks as the day wears on, by mid-afternoon, we're going to be feeling spectacularly blah—in the grip of a slump from which no amount of coffee or sugar can extract us. Meanwhile, the expense of all this physiological overtime effort will be accruing. We can expect to see:

- Rising markers of inflammation

- Increased blood pressure

- Imbalanced blood sugar and insulin response

- Higher cholesterol

- Lowered immunity

- Imbalanced neurotransmitters

- Declining mental capacity

- Gaps in memory

- Disrupted digestion

- Imbalanced acid-alkaline levels

- Slowed metabolism

- Increased moodiness and emotional reactivity

- Increased sugar and carb cravings

- Diminished communication and relational skills

- Decreased observational capacity

- Declining motor skills

Additionally, as a result of these operational downgrades, we incur a wide range of secondary costs and risks:

- We can't think straight, so our error rate increases, our reading comprehension is reduced, and our productivity plummets.

- Our peripheral vision narrows, so we miss things we'd normally notice.

- Our creativity declines, so we have a harder time coming up with good ideas and solutions.

- Our physical coordination is reduced, so we type more slowly, produce more typos and transposed numbers; our likelihood of stubbing a toe, spilling our coffee, or having more serious accidents rises precipitously.

- Our cravings for sugar and refined carbs incline us to eat a bunch of junk food that further contributes to inflammation and blood-sugar imbalances, tanking our energy and resilience, and leaving us feeling like crap.

- Disruption of normal sleep patterns and decline in sleep quality further reduce our effectiveness, while further undermining mood, immunity, and cognitive performance.

In other words, as we skip ultradian rhythm breaks, we get diminishing returns and escalating risks on every level. And the more ultradian rhythm breaks we skip, the worse the damage becomes. That's why, by the end of the day, so many people are husks of their former selves, walking bundles of deadened and frayed nerves. It's why so many people get home from a hard day's work only to fall on the couch in a heap, devour a bunch of unhealthy food, have multiple alcoholic drinks, or wind up in peevish exchanges with their loved ones.

Hormonally speaking, it's also why a lot of working couples wind up having less sex (and enjoying sex less) than they'd like. But we'll come back to that later. Because believe it or not, this all gets worse. If we ignore our ultradian rhythms for days, weeks, or months at a time, the accumulated damage and distress become more tangible, producing a variety of nasty potential results:

- Flaring of inflammatory symptoms, like rashes, cold sores and lymph-related bumps

- Back and neck pain, headaches

- Stomach pain, digestive distress

- Hormonal imbalances

- Brain damage and memory loss

- Mood imbalances

- Alterations to DNA (activating disease-causing polymorphisms)

- Accumulation of fat stores, especially around the belly

- Unconscious obsessive-compulsive behaviors like nail biting, cuticle picking, cheek or lip biting, hair pulling, and scratching

- Accelerated aging

- Hair loss and thinning ... and pretty much all of the things you'll find on the Weird Symptom Checklist (see chapter 4)

Eventually, the inflamed and diminished state of the body-mind (caused by the destructive effects of delayed maintenance, repair, and detoxification) can set the stage for serious conditions like heart disease, type 2 diabetes, autoimmune disorders, migraines, arthritis, depression, Alzheimer's, and more.

I know it might seem tough to believe that all of these awful things could result from something as seemingly insignificant as some missed rest breaks. And, of course, many of the same negative effects can be created or exacerbated by other factors, including poor nutrition, environmental toxins, infectious diseases, and so on.

But when you think about it objectively, it makes sense that extended ultradian-rhythm mismanagement can play a huge role in degrading our health, sanity, and general well-being: Whenever you repeatedly overdrive and under-maintain *any* system, it tends to fail.

We've heard a great deal about the importance of sleep in the past few years. We now understand that our bodies accomplish the majority of their intensive repair and biochemical rebalancing work while we slumber. When it looks like we're doing nothing, our bodies are actually doing some of the most important tasks imaginable.

Well, ultradian rhythm breaks are like "sleep snacks"—not naps, per se, but similar in their potential to return a tired and depleted body to higher function.

The problem is that we've got some serious cultural programming to overcome here, not just about sleep, but about rest and recovery and self-care in general. The American work ethic is all about non-stop activity and determination. It has a long history of glorifying acts of hard work, self-sacrifice, suffering, and endurance. We like the idea of pushing through, hanging in there, just doing it, and grinding away until something is done. We tend to think of taking a break as being a sign of weakness, a sissy-quitter thing to do, a surefire way to tank our productivity or otherwise undermine our value.

Research says otherwise. A lot of research.[33] But since research can be boring to read and tough to remember, I like to offer a couple of helpful metaphors that might help drive the key points of the research home.

The Ultradian Car

Think about your body as a combustion-engine vehicle you're driving down the road. As it burns fuel to power its forward motion, the vehicle produces exhaust. Except in this case, the vehicle's tailpipe is venting directly into your car's interior.

When enough biochemical and neurological smog accumulates in there, the air gets thick. You start getting light-headed and nauseous from the pollution. It becomes difficult to see through the haze and increasingly difficult for you to think straight.

In order for your body to get all the junk out of your system and in order for your brain to effectively process all the random particulate-bits of data that are floating around and clogging up your synaptic circuitry, your whole vehicular system needs a break.

If you pull over, turn the engine off, roll the windows down, and let some fresh air blow in, everything clears out pretty quickly. Once you're feeling good (and can see the windshield again), you can get back on the road for another stint. But stay in that smoggy, fume-infested car for too long, and, well, let's just say you're going to get nowhere fast.

The Ultradian Shop

Think of your body-mind as a busy retail store that's being overrun with excited customers, all wanting to peruse, try on, and purchase things. Some are lined up to buy gift certificates and place special orders; others want things wrapped and shipped; others have returns and exchanges.

After a couple hours of this high level of activity, the shop is a mess, inventory is running low, the credit card machine is on the fritz, transactions are being processed by hand, and boxes and paperwork are piled up all over the place. The clerks are starting to make mistakes; the customers are getting snippy and impatient.

All of this creates slow-downs, confusion, and conflicts that make the store less efficient, less pleasant, and less profitable. Stressed out and overworked, some of the staff are peevish, in tears, and on the verge of quitting. Once-enthusiastic customers are complaining and starting to post negative reviews on Yelp.

At this point, a smart manager would hang a little "please come back shortly" sign on the door, giving the staff a chance to catch their breath, restock the shelves, tidy up the shop, reboot the credit card machine, and so on. About twenty minutes later, they can let the customers back in to a clean, beautiful, well-stocked store, and provide them with a terrific shopping experience.

Okay, you get the idea. But by now you may also be thinking: Hey, wait, isn't this what coffee breaks are for?

In a way, yes. For people whose focused efforts begin at eight or nine in the morning, the typical times for ultradian troughs to hit are mid-morning, midday, and mid-afternoon. It's no accident that those are the same times many people automatically reach for caffeinated drinks, refined carbs, and cigarettes.

While these solutions can provide temporary relief (refined carbs and caffeine work by forcing the system into a momentary energy spike; cigarettes by blunting feelings of emotional stress), they browbeat the body into overriding its own intelligent ultradian programming. They also establish unhealthy dependencies. Worse, by elevating inflammation, adding toxic burdens, and triggering immune-system responses, they impinge on the physiological recovery and repair opportunity the body and brain are so desperate for.

Accordingly, while getting up from your task to go get said coffee or sugar or cigarette might serve some ultradian purpose, the inputs themselves tend to have a predominantly negative effect. They might give you the impression that you've gotten yourself through an energetic slump, but they don't do much to return the body and brain to a state of optimal function. For that, you need a real, honest-to-goodness ultradian rhythm break.

So, how does one take a proper URB? Well, there is a wide spectrum of options with varying levels of return. The best way, according to scientific research (much of which has been done by the U.S. Department of Defense), is to cease all action and directed thought, lie down (preferably in a dark, quiet room or with a light-blocking eye mask and earplugs on board), and try to fall asleep.

Now, obviously, that's not going to be doable for most folks who work a regular job or who are in school, surrounded by children, or in the midst of busy public spaces at the time the need for a URB hits. Fortunately, you don't have to sleep (or even lie down) for your URBs in order to have them count. Reclining, leaning, and moving calmly (e.g., walking, doing yoga, stretching) are all good options. The main thing is to let your body relax, to get out of whatever static position or posture it's been in, and to let your mind wander, slow, and be calm.

Ultimately, any mental and physical break—or even a shift of focus to something different and less demanding—is better than nothing. And any quality time spent taking a URB better than none. Here's a quick recap of why and how to take your URBs ...

Ultradian Rhythm Break (URB) Basics

WHY?

- Upgrade your energy, focus, capacity, and resilience.

- Rebalance blood sugar, neurotransmitters, and hormones.

- Support body-wide detoxification and repair.

- Ward off unhealthy cravings and mood swings.

- Boost and safeguard immunity.

- Improve productivity and creative problem solving.

- Capture big insights, ideas, and aha moments.

- Create space for healthy nourishment, activity, and social connections.

- Reinforce the practice of respecting your body's hardwired systems.

HOW?

- Start noticing that throughout the course of each day, your body moves through a repeating, oscillating energy cycle, rising to an energy peak over the course of hour and a half to two hours, and then dropping into an energy trough that lasts about twenty minutes.

- Know that these low-energy troughs are your friend and that they have a purpose: Getting you to take a physical and mental break so that your body can repair, rebalance, replenish, reorganize, and detoxify its core systems.

- Be on the lookout for signals that you need URBs. They include fatigue, brain fog, loss of focus and productivity, yawning, fidgeting, difficulty keeping your eyes open, irritation, hunger, thirst, clumsiness, increasing errors, and any kind of bathroom urge (when you need to go, *go!*).

- Watch for ultradian troughs to strike in the midmorning and midafternoon (within two hours of starting work and within two hours after lunch). At the first signs of depletion (or ideally, before), stop what you are doing and take a break: Twenty minutes is ideal, but any break (even five or ten minutes) is better than nothing. The longer and more chill your break is, the more repair and replenishing work your body will do.

- Give your body and mind a chance to shift gears. If you've been sitting still, move. If you've been moving, sit still. If you've been focusing intensely, let your brain shut down.

- Doing puttering manual tasks is okay (fill your stapler, empty the trash), but avoid any intensive demands or distractions, including the use of electronics and digital media.

- Consider setting a timed alert that prompts you to assess your state of energy and focus every ninety minutes or so. Once you become adept at noticing your own energetic rhythms (review the first Nonconformist Competency, Amplified Awareness), you'll no longer need an external alert.

Optional URB Activities

Feel free to combine one or more of the following (based on what your body craves) for a total of ten to twenty minutes, or for however long you can manage:

- Hit the restroom (even if you don't think you have to go).

- Get a drink of water or cup of tea and enjoy drinking it slowly.

- Grab a healthy snack (avoid refined carbs and sugars) and eat it away from your desk and while not doing anything productive, demanding, or attention-distracting.

- Get outside and walk calmly (looking around you, not at your smartphone).

- Try one or more of the Three Walks exercises described in chapter 18.

- Stare into space or out the window, seeing if you notice an interesting shape, color, or scene.

- Close your eyes and meditate or do deep breathing.

- Sit on a curb or bench and let your mind wander for a while.

- Walk around the building looking for things you never noticed before.

- Visit with a colleague or friend, expressing interest or positive feelings.

- Listen to a guided meditation or piece of calming music.

- Do a little restorative yoga (shivasana is highly recommended).

- Do a mindless task, like refilling your stapler or cleaning out your purse or a drawer.

- Run a simple or pleasant errand (e.g., picking up flowers, shopping for a gift).

- Rub some lotion or balm into your hands, cuticles, and elbows.

- Waft some aromatherapy oils or flower essences around your space.

- Call a loved one to say hi or to express love and appreciation.

- Visualize how you want the rest of your day or evening to go.

- Make a quick list of things you are grateful for.

- Reflect on a list of your core values and notice which ones have been in play today.

- Ask yourself what you're hankering for and do something to honor that.

- Consider the body position you've been in for the last hour, and assume some contrasting position. If you've been leaning forward, stretch backward. If you've been sitting, stand up or lie down. If you've been still, move about. If you've been looking down, look up. If you've been focusing your eyes close-up, look far away.

What you *don't* want to do is more of whatever you've been doing for the past couple hours, especially if that's looking at some kind of screen. You need a shift of gears, a reboot, a change of scene. The main thing you need to know is this:

> The more you understand and respect your own ultradian rhythms, the more capable you'll be of getting the best from your body and mind.

The other thing to know is that since *almost nobody* knows anything about ultradian rhythms or URBs, very few workplaces, schools, or organized events do anything to respect or accommodate them. Which means that the minute you begin to observe them yourself, you'll probably be seen as a bit of an oddball. That pretty much goes with the Healthy Deviant territory, I'm afraid. Might as well get used to it.

On the bright side, when you explain the logic of your URBs to people (remember the car and store metaphors?), they will often wind up nodding along with you and saying, "Wow, yeah. That makes perfect sense!" Sometimes, once they've tried taking these breaks for themselves, they'll wind up thanking you and telling you that you've changed their life. And then you can say, "Hey, if you like Ultradian Rhythm Breaks, I bet you would love my Nighttime Wind-Down Ritual...."

The Case of the Beanbag-Chair Napper

A few years back, in a workshop I taught in Silicon Valley (at 1440 Multiversity), one of the participants was an executive at a leading accounting-software company. Let's call him Bill. After seeing my presentation on ultradian rhythms, Bill told me that he had been getting a lot of pressure from members of his group to "come down on" a particular software engineer (let's call him Joe) who was famous for taking naps on a beanbag chair in his cube in the middle of the day.

Joe's coworkers were apparently not wild about his napping on the job. They kept taking pictures of him asleep on the beanbag and sending them, by way of complaint, to Bill. Bill told me he'd been feeling increasingly pressured to reprimand Joe over the past few months, but seeing my presentation was making him reconsider whether this was, in fact, a behavior he wanted to discourage. Perhaps, he thought, Joe knew something that his coworkers didn't.

I asked him how Joe's productivity and creativity were relative to the rest of his group. He told me that, interestingly, Joe was among his best, most creative, and productive employees. He also sounded like a pretty nice, fun guy—a classic Healthy Deviant. I told Bill that I thought he had his answer. Rather than reprimanding Joe, I thought he might be wise to "make an example of him" in a *good* way, holding him up as a model of productive self-management and efficiency.

Ultradian Timing

Until you get really good at recognizing and respecting your body's ultradian signals, it's best to set a timer that will remind you to take a break (or at least check in with yourself) every ninety minutes or so. I love the low-tech simplicity of the analog devices made by the Time Timer company (which I learned about in Jake Knapp and John Zeratsky's terrific book, *Make Time: How to Focus on What Matters Every Day* (Random House, 2018), but you can use any timer you like, including an app on your cell phone.

When the timer goes off, ask yourself, "How am I feeling right now?"

> **If you're feeling great, terrific.** Take the break anyway, and you'll be on course to enjoy that energy all day long. Once you're in a groove, you can experiment with extending your work sprints slightly, but don't go beyond two hours, or you'll see declining returns.

> **If you're feeling a bit fatigued, spacey, hungry, thirsty, or distracted, ask yourself:** "Have I been feeling this way for a while?" If so, you'll want to set your breaks to happen a bit earlier, or shift your break intervals to be more frequent.

There are some schools of thought (like the Pomodoro Method) that suggest taking breaks more frequently, like once an hour or even every twenty-five minutes. It's up to you to sort out which rhythms work best for your physiology and life. But for most people, taking a URB for ten to twenty minutes every hour and a half is a great place to start.

Alert and Reminder Tips

There are many different types of apps and alarm mechanisms that make it easy to establish timed intervals for productive (or meditative) sprints. As noted, I'm a fan of Time Timers (TimeTimer.com). But the built-in timing functions on your watch, phone, computer, or even a simple kitchen timer will do. Just strive to find an alarm that isn't too jarring and a timer that's fast and easy for you to set and reset. To date, I haven't found a particular app for this that I adore (I'm actually thinking about creating one, so if you're an app developer and want to partner on that, let me know!). Because I am nearsighted and don't enjoy punching the tiny keys on my phone, I sometimes simply tell Siri, "Remind me to take a break in ninety minutes." That seems to work fine.

It doesn't really matter how you go about timing your breaks, but it *does* matter that you physically time them, at least for a while. Once you become adept at noticing your body's "I need a break!" signals, you may find that your body is, in fact, doing all the timing for you and that you no longer need an alarm at all.

One thing you probably *will* want a timer for, at least for now, is organizing your final URB of the day, which is so important that it qualifies as a Renegade Ritual of its own—the Nighttime Wind-Down.

For now, just remember this:

How We've Been Told We're Supposed to Work

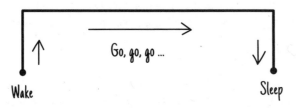

How We Actually Work

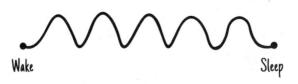

Nighttime Wind-Down

Finish each day and be done with it.
You have done what you could;
some blunders and absurdities have crept in;
forget them as soon as you can.
Tomorrow is a new day;
you shall begin it serenely and with too high a spirit
to be encumbered with your old nonsense.

—RALPH WALDO EMERSON

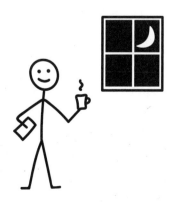

After a long day of go-go-go activity, many people come home to an evening's worth of equally intense demands or, alternately, to numbing entertainments. Some continue work tasks late into the evening or do home- and family-related tasks straight until they go to bed. Others watch television or movies or play games to zone out, often putting sleep off for hours beyond a healthy bedtime.

They then fall into bed exhausted—but still wired—and have trouble falling asleep. Or they fall asleep only to wake again a few hours later, sometimes as the result of cycling worries, sometimes from the effects of alcoholic beverages they imbibed as a way to relax, detach, and put the day behind them.

The human nervous system wasn't designed for binary on-off operations, and the amount of adrenaline and cortisol produced during a too-busy or too-stressful day can pose a huge barrier to proper sleep—unless it is allowed to taper off and be replaced by pro-relaxation biochemicals (like melatonin and oxytocin) prior to retiring. Instituting a regular evening ritual helps accomplish this goal, preparing the body and mind for a good night's rest, and providing a conscious conclusion to the day.

Nighttime Wind-Down Basics

WHY?

- Allow for mental and physical "deceleration"—the slowing and settling down of the body-mind's complex, interconnected systems and signaling mechanisms.

- Set the stage for high-quality sleep by encouraging an advantageous mix and balance of neurotransmitters and hormones.

- Conquer insomnia and mid-sleep waking patterns.

- Optimize body's tissue-repair window and capacity.

- Set yourself up for success the next day by optimizing overnight energy regeneration.

- Support healthy circadian and ultradian rhythm cycles.

- Reduce inflammation, compromised metabolism, and hormone imbalance.

- Improve recovery from stress, trauma, and fitness activity.

- Improve romantic connection and create windows for intimacy.

HOW?

- Starting about an hour before bedtime (set an alert to remind you), begin winding down the active part of your day and preparing for sleep.

- Close down all work and shut off all screen-based devices and entertainments.

- Shift the energy and mood in your home: Lower house lights and sound, put on some relaxing music, or just enjoy the silence.

- Make yourself a warm, non-caffeinated beverage (like herbal tea or warm water) to sip as you complete the final actions of your day.

- Do your Evening Ablutions (see below) or other self-care activities in a calm, pleasant, ritualized way.

- Prepare your bedroom for sleep, making sure all light sources are completely darkened or blocked and the room temperature is lowered.

- Once you get into bed, do so with the intention of going to sleep. But allow for space *between* wake and sleep. Remember, the body operates in oscillating curves and waves, not binary on-off switches.

What the Heck Are Evening Ablutions?

The word *ablution* is an old-fashioned term that describes a ritualized act of self-washing or anointing with cleansing oils. This, I have found, is a great way to go about one's morning and evening wash-up and dental-care routines—the things most of us do a couple times a day anyway.

As you lather, scrub, rinse, moisturize, brush, and floss, intentionally slow down. Touch your face and body with reverence and care; assume an "ablution" consciousness. Make whatever you are doing a mindful self-grooming ritual, not just another perfunctory to-do. Make it a sacred rite rather than a rushed obligation. Take care of your body like it matters, like you love and value it just the way it is, and you will find it responds with relaxation, appreciation, and pleasure—not a bad way to head toward sleep.

Optional Wind-Down Activities

- As you are concluding your day's projects, note any uncompleted tasks so you can get them off your brain without fear of losing track of them.

- Neatly stack your work. Review your next day's schedule and gather anything you'll need to take with you.

- As you turn your devices off, also set them to charge.

- Make sure your car keys, wallet, purse, and other bags are where you want them for the next day.

- After lowering the house lights as low as you practically can, consider lighting a few candles.

- Do a quick walk-through of the kitchen and your Morning Minutes practice area. Clear off any surfaces you've dirtied or cluttered up during your evening meal or activities.

- Get into your pajamas or strip down to your birthday suit. Soften the light in your bedroom or light candles. Waft some aromatherapy oil around. Rub a little moisturizing balm on your hands, feet, elbows.

- Look for and block any ambient lights or glowing displays, including small lights from smoke alarms and electronic thermostats.

- If you read before bed, read only from paper books, not electronic tablets. Steer clear of scary or distressing subjects, and avoid professional reading. Keep reading lights as low as tolerable.

- If you're doing the Healthy Deviant Adventure program, reserve a few minutes to review your Daily Deviance Journal Pages.

- Reflect on how your day went. Picture yourself back at your Morning Minutes practice area, and recall setting your intentions (do you remember what they were or how they played out?).

- Review any bright spots (positive moments, experiences or accomplishments that stand out) or areas of challenge; take stock of your blessings and feel your gratitude.

- Snuggle, love-up, or just be with yourself or your sleeping partner. If you have a partner, consider sharing some warm fuzzy thought or appreciation with them.

- When you are ready, turn off or blow out any remaining light sources.

- Take a big, deep breath; relax all your muscles (try first tensing and then relaxing any that don't seem to want to let go); then decide to release the day (see "A Mantra to Sleep On," below).

- Know that you have been enough, done enough. Now, it's time to rest, repair, recover—so that your body and mind can wake up ready to take on tomorrow.

A Mantra to Sleep On

If you have difficulty letting the day go, or you have a mind that stays active long after you lie down, consider adopting a bedtime mantra (one you can repeat silently or aloud) as a way of confirming—for both your body and mind—that you are ready to relax and sleep.

For example, my older sister, who used to work at a domestic-abuse shelter and often came home stressed by the stories she'd heard, sometimes used the mantra "I am safe and cozy" to help her drift off. It worked well enough for her that she shared it with her clients at the shelter, and many told her they found it helpful in unwinding the fight-or-flight mindset they inhabited by default.

Interestingly, even though my sister no longer works at the shelter, her body-mind became so well trained to respond positively to her sleep mantra from that era that she sometimes still uses it today.

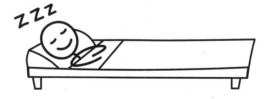

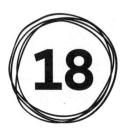

Healthy Deviant Survival Skills

Extinction is the rule. Survival is the exception.

—CARL SAGAN

Canvass that rare breed of individuals who have maintained both their health and their happiness over a long period of time, and you'll find they have some interesting things in common: Not some inborn gift of willpower or moral superiority, but a characteristic set of healthy-person skills. As noted in chapter 11, I think of them as new era survival skills. These skills make it vastly easier to make conscious, self-preserving choices, to maintain healthy mindsets, and to ward off the siren songs of the Unhealthy Default Reality (UDR).

Such skills are not widely taught in our culture, but they can be learned by anyone with enough moxie and desire to develop them. You can go about acquiring your Healthy Deviant Survival Skills at whatever pace (and in whatever order) you choose. The specific skills you need will depend on your current circumstances, including your health status, stage of life, and the goals or desires you are pursuing now.

The importance of the Nonconformist Competencies (Amplified Awareness, Preemptive Repair, and Continuous Growth and Learning) remains constant, but the current focus within each of those competencies will naturally shift over time.

To get at the skills you might currently most benefit from developing in each area of competence, consider these questions:

- **In the realm of Amplified Awareness:** What are you becoming aware of in the domain of yourself, your circumstances, tendencies, and triggers? What is capturing your attention, and why?

- **In the realm of Preemptive Repair:** In what ways are you seeking to strengthen and repair yourself, to become less reactive and more resilient? What aspects of your body, mind, and heart have been sending you distress signals or signs of depletion?

- **In the realm of Continuous Growth and Learning:** What knowledge, skills, or capacities are you feeling most in need of or curious about right now? What abilities, if you had them, would make the biggest difference in your life?

In answering those questions, you will naturally zero in on some implied Healthy Deviant skills—things that, if you knew how to do or pursue them, would make you stronger, more gratified, and more resilient to the Unhealthy Default Reality.

The scientific literature spells out some clear advice on what you can do to avoid getting worn down (keep your blood sugar stable, don't take on too many difficult things at once). And it offers plenty of obvious counsel on how to rebuild your stores once they are depleted (eat healthy food, exercise, and sleep). But it doesn't often (or at least often enough, in my opinion) address *how you can go about doing any of those things in the context of the UDR.*

Over the years, having delved deep into both a lot of scientific studies and a vast trove of self-help literature, and having tried a lot of that advice out myself, here's an amalgamation of the advice I've found most useful:[34]

- **Don't push your luck:** Whenever possible, restrict the UDR's access to you. Don't spend time randomly browsing around on the internet or in shopping centers "for fun." Steer clear of fast-food strips and food courts where engineered-to-be-irresistible smells grab you. Avoid letting always-on conventional media play in the background of your life. Turn off video screens and turn down audio volume whenever and wherever you can (not just in your own home, but in taxi cabs, on planes, in waiting rooms, and so on). Avoid conventional magazine racks at bookstores and supermarkets. Don't browse social feeds that nurse your self-doubt or trigger unhealthy obsessions.

- **Don't count on the UDR to solve problems for you:** Keep solutions low on the consumer index and within your current means. Buying into expensive meal-replacement shakes, food-delivery programs, and studio-based workouts, for example, is probably not a great solution if they are not something you can afford for the long haul. No fitness device or fat-melting contraption you order off the internet is going to resolve the deeper challenges of choosing to be a healthy person in an unhealthy world.

- **Build momentum through easy wins:** Build your mojo and willpower muscles with small-scale self-regulation exercises before you take on huge or scary ones.[35] Practice on easier things first. Experiment with self-regulation in situations that are not your kryptonite scenarios (which, for most people, include diet and exercise). Do some of the things you *can* do before trying to do one or more things you think you *can't*. If you can't give up your morning donut, but you can make your bed before you leave the house, do that. If you can start meditating more easily than you can start swinging kettlebells, do that. Keep the power of what is known as "positive spillover" on your side.

Please Don't Freak Out

In just a moment, I'm going to hit you with a long list of Healthy Deviant Tendencies. These are areas of skill, awareness, and preference that Healthy Deviants are inclined to develop and leverage to a greater degree than most others. But before you read that list and start beating up on yourself for not having already embraced or mastered all of them, I want to emphasize that all you really need to do right now is notice which of them (if any) is currently calling to you and potentially within reach. Notice what pops. Notice what sings. Notice what you are already doing and what you might feel most interested in doing next. The rest will come in time.

Here's a handy chart to help you decide where, among all of the healthy choices in the world, you will probably have the most success in focusing your attention.

Where to Start?

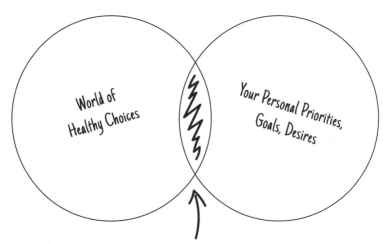

World of Healthy Choices

Your Personal Priorities, Goals, Desires

Healthy Stuff You Are Energized to Do <u>Now</u>

Healthy Deviant Tendencies

Healthy Deviants are a diverse lot. They don't walk in lock step with anyone else, and as individuals, they all manage their daily choices differently, because they do what works for them. Some eat meat; some don't.[36] Some are gym rats; others bookish. They come in all shapes and sizes, in all races, genders, and ages, and inhabit all sorts of locations on the political spectrum.

Unfortunately, because we live in a society that has made healthy choices comparatively expensive, inconvenient, and inaccessible, Healthy Deviants with fewer financial resources often encounter much greater barriers in accessing their preferred choices. So as noted, this is *not* an even playing field. Even so, there are some skills, wisdom, and tendencies that many Healthy Deviants have in common:

- They highly value their health and will, whenever possible, prioritize it above most other things.

- They tend to take a systems approach to health, seeing it as a whole-life enterprise, and seeing all of the pieces of the body-mind puzzle as inherently connected.

- They tend to be constant learners, continually expanding their healthy skill sets.

- They tend to focus on the fundamentals first: Stay sane, eat real food, drink water, move your body, get good sleep, surround yourself with good people, do what makes you happy.

- They understand that what works for a friend or family member may not work for them, and that what worked for them ten years ago may not work for them now.

- They may share what they know with others but are disinclined to put pressure on others to do precisely what they are doing.

Despite their diversity, Healthy Deviants tend to approach a lot of the choices related to their health and well-being in some characteristic ways—not just in terms of nutrition and movement, but also around sleep, stress, self-image, how they relate to media, how they interpret science, and how they approach health care.

For example, Healthy Deviants tend to be far more likely than "normal" people to do things like those in the list that follows. But again, please keep in mind that this list is intended to be *descriptive,* not *prescriptive.* Frankly, not a single Healthy Deviant person whom I know (including me) does *all* these things *all* of the time, so please don't fret or panic if you aren't currently and consistently doing them all yourself.

Food and Eating

Healthy Deviants tend to:

- Care a lot about what they eat, and enjoy eating, but don't spend a lot of time obsessing about it.

- Eat mostly whole, natural, unprocessed foods most of the time.

- Practice conscious eating, refuse to "diet," and avoid any approach to eating that involves counting calories or points.

- Know how to make simple, good-tasting food at home and where to find healthy whole-foods away from home (to the extent they are available).

- Eat a lot of non-starchy, brightly colored vegetables.

- Prefer local, organic, seasonal, grass-fed, wild-caught, and sustainably and humanely raised foods to the extent they are available and affordable.

- Moderate their intake of grains and starches based on their current energy needs.

- Avoid gluten-containing grains and gluten-containing processed food products, regardless of their celiac status, if they've found they feel better not eating them.

- Avoid low-fat dairy, understanding that full-fat dairy is better for you (assuming you can tolerate dairy).

- Recognize that vegetarian and "plant-based" diets can be unhealthy if not composed, in large part, of actual plants (as opposed to grains, flours, starches), and if they do not also contain adequate and appropriate combinations of proteins, healthy fats, vitamins, minerals, and phytonutrients.

- Eat the same way in private as in public; don't fear eating-disapproval from others.

- Understand that the food that works for their friends and family may not work for them.

- Avoid most processed foods, fast foods, and junk foods, including products (like breakfast cereals) where flours, industrial oils, and sugars are among the first ingredients.

- Avoid foods with chemical additives, preservatives, flavorings, and other potentially irritating or toxic ingredients.

- Rarely consume candy, pastry, soft drinks (regular or diet), sweetened coffee drinks, energy drinks, sports drinks, and sweet alcoholic beverages.

- Reject low-fat, reduced-fat, diet, zero-calorie, and lite foods in favor of their less processed, full-fat, and naturally sweetened counterparts.

- Avoid meal-replacement shakes and liquid diets (except as required for short-term medical protocols).

- Learn and respect their food intolerances or sensitivities; experiment to find out what does and does not agree with them.

- Know that the most common dietary irritants are gluten, dairy, sugar, soy, eggs, wheat, corn, tree nuts, and alcohol.

- Reject the idea of "cheat" days in favor of just eating in ways that please them and feel good to them most of the time. Periodically enjoy some less-healthy foods just for fun—without guilt or anxiety.

Sleep and Recovery

Healthy Deviants tend to:

- Make sleep and rest a huge priority.

- Go to bed earlier and rise earlier than most.

- Decline or cancel social plans in favor of getting enough sleep.

- Prefer to wind down before bed with relaxing, low-key activities.

- Lower house lights and turn off blue-light displays well before bedtime.

- Not keep televisions or other entertainment-oriented electronics in their bedrooms.

- Not bring work in their bedrooms.

- Keep their sleeping environments cool (under 68 degrees), dark, and as quiet as possible.

- Block all the light coming into their bedrooms at night, and cover all light-emitting displays, including digital-clock, thermostat, and smoke-alarm lights.

- Avoid eating big meals or drinking alcoholic beverages close to bedtime.

- Avoid dependence on pharmaceutical or recreational drugs as sleep aids.

- Strive to create a bedroom "haven" environment by reducing clutter, mess, and distraction.

- Keep allergy-causing and noise-creating pets out of the bedroom.

- Choose natural, breathable, non-toxic bedding materials when possible.

Exercise

Healthy Deviants tend to:

- See physical movement as essential to both their physical and mental-emotional health.

- Build a variety of movement opportunities and active breaks into their days.

- Pursue forms of activity or exercise they enjoy and find interesting (which they may or may not think about as "working out").

- Be more focused on building strength, flexibility, agility, fitness, and body-awareness than on losing weight or achieving a particular look or body composition.

- Be willing to try lots of things to see what they like, but are not beholden to fitness fads or trends.

- Enjoy moving outdoors when they can and seek to spend some time outside each day.

- Be likely to stand for at least part of long presentations, conferences, flights, and other occasions when others remain seated.

- Be inclined to take stairs when they are available.

- Prefer to carry their own grocery bags, luggage, and other heavy things.

- Embrace some active leisure activities or hobbies and enjoy spending time with friends in ways that involve moving.

- Hugely value their mobility and see movement as something they *get* to do, rather than something they have to do.

Stress Management

Healthy Deviants tend to:

- Recognize when they are under excessive stress and take steps to reduce or manage it.

- Be willing to renegotiate commitments if they realize they are no longer going to work for them.

- Use meditation, mindfulness, yoga, cognitive behavioral therapy, and related practices to reduce reactivity and manage emotional responses and negative thinking.

- Use good communication skills to lower stress in relationships.

- Avoid lying, cheating, stealing, and scheming.

- Do not tolerate protracted periods of conflict and anger in their relationships; seek to resolve and transform them in constructive, positive, proactive ways.

- Adopt a "learner" (growth) vs. "judger" (fixed) mindset in resolving problems.

- Seek help from a therapist, counselor, or coach when they feel overwhelmed or unable to work through a problem on their own.

- Make time for pleasure, fun, and social activity.

- Surround themselves with a small group of close friends and loved ones.

Self-Image

Healthy Deviants tend to:

- Find plenty of things to like and love about their body at any size and shape.

- Don't bad-talk their own appearance.

- Don't panic if their weight fluctuates up or down a bit.

- Notice if their weight changes significantly, and become interested in why.

- Avoid comparing their bodies to others'—and recognize when they do.

- Do not respond to hype about "perfecting" their body parts.

- Find themselves sexy and feel good in their own skin.

- Carry themselves with confidence and take pride in their healthy appearance without obsessing over it.

- Refuse to spend a lot of time ogling the pictures in beauty or health and fitness magazines.

- Recognize they are living in a world where the hyper-perfected models of beauty are unrealistic.

Media Literacy

Healthy Deviants tend to:

- Limit their exposure to mass media, social media, and all forms of "always on" media.

- Create "sacred spaces" in their lives and environments where all forms of media are turned off.

- Be more interested in what is going on in their own lives than the lives of fictional characters and celebrities.

- Avoid conventional health and fitness magazines, or read them with a skeptical eye.

- Recognize that virtually all photos of models and celebrities are radically retouched (after hours of preparation, styling, and perfecting by a crew of professional hair, makeup, wardrobe, and lighting specialists).

- Realize that the church-and-state line separating editorial content and advertising is now almost nonexistent.

- Understand that in virtually all environments where you are not paying for content, you (meaning your eyes, ears, and mindshare) are "the product"—the target for advertising or a source for tracked data.

- Get their media from multiple, reputable sources, rather than one or two fringe outlets.

- Know the difference between real news and "fake news."

- Fact-check questionable claims and know how to follow the money in tracing the motivations behind powerful and wealthy special interests.

- Know what "astroturfing" is, how it works, why powerful corporate and political interests do it, and why otherwise reputable experts might get called quacks, fear-mongers, and racketeers (or worse) as a result.

Science Literacy

Healthy Deviants tend to:

- Know that scientific results can be skewed or misreported or undermined as the result of industry interference or researcher bias.

- Be skeptical of sensational scientific headlines, knowing that the media often vastly simplifies or totally mischaracterizes study findings.

- Question reported research findings that make outsized claims.

- Be interested, when evaluating scientific research, not just in the study size and whether the research was on animals or humans, but also the methods used, how researchers drew their conclusions, and whether the researchers had any conflicts of interest.

- Mistrust interpretations of science (and critiques of science) that come from powerful industries with vested interests or people with evident axes to grind.

- Follow the money in investigating the potential motives behind questionable studies and reports.

- Understand the difference between causation and correlation, knowing that much of the research purporting to prove causal effects draws on correlations that can be explained by other means.

- Understand that while randomized clinical trials are the "gold standard" of science, they are not necessarily the only evidence to follow.

- Know the limitations of nutrition studies, many of which are based on self-reported data or very short-term feeding windows, not long-term, real-life, complex eating scenarios.

- Consider how specific lab-based studies might apply (or not) to their real-life circumstances and selves (studies done on middle-aged, sedentary, white men eating standard American diets, for example, may not apply equally to children, older people, athletes, women, or people of color, or to people *not* eating standard American diets).

- Look for the patterns in studies over time and seek corroborating information rather than shifting their entire approach based on a one-off study result.

- Be inclined to experiment on themselves and conduct their own "N of 1" studies (studies in which they are the sole subject) in order to see how specific approaches or interventions will work for them.

Health-Care Literacy

Healthy Deviants tend to:

- See themselves as responsible for their own well-being, and to self-direct many aspects of their health care.

- Pay close attention to signals their body is in distress.

- Rely on the conventional medical system as little as possible, except in case of acute injuries or life-threatening events.

- Be interested in books, videos, and educational programs related to health.

- Seek out the mental and emotional health support they need, to the extent it is accessible and affordable to them.

- Prefer to avoid prescription drugs and elective medical procedures whenever possible.

- See food as medicine and be willing to adjust their diets for improved health.

- Understand that most conventional doctors receive little training in nutrition or lifestyle medicine.

- Have a posse of healing practitioners and advisors whom they turn to for ongoing support with health challenges.

- Be willing to pay out of pocket for preferred health-care services (to the extent they can find and afford them).

What You Don't Know (Yet) Will Save You

I realize that seems like a whole lot of stuff to know and master, and it is. But, as noted, you don't have to (and really can't) wade into all of it all at once. You also don't have to do it all or do any of it 100 percent of the time in order to be an unusually healthy person or qualify as a Healthy Deviant.

If you're interested in expanding your healthy-person skills, consider making a little checklist of the top five areas of capacity you don't yet possess (gathered from the above lists or the top of your mind), and that seem like they'd have the biggest positive impact if you developed them.

1. _____

2. _____

3. _____

4. _____

5. _____

Next, select the top three of those and place them in order of your willingness to begin learning or embracing them right now.

1. _____

2. _____

3. _____

Finally, take the top item, and identify two easy, painless things you could do in the span of less than three minutes to even *slightly* expand your knowledge base or motivation on that subject. Here are just a few possible options: Doing a quick web search, watching a short video, or identifying a good book on the subject; calling a friend who has the skill or habit and asking them how they developed it; starting a clipping file for references and resources on the topic; or envisioning yourself masterfully doing the thing in question.

Jot down your two easy-to-do-things below (if you can't think of anything, feel free to copy down one or more of the ideas listed above).

1. _____

2. _____

Next, take the next sixty seconds to *begin* taking action on *one* of those things now—meaning right this minute. Just set this book aside for a moment, and even if you can't complete the action, use the span of one full minute to do something in the service of your goal.

Find Your Next Step

Okay, how does it feel to have done something, even a tiny thing, to build your healthy-living mojo? Do you feel remotely interested in going further with this task or in taking a crack at the second small-scale action you listed above?

Now, take a look back at the longer list of five things you started with. Can you imagine approaching any of them in this same way—little piece by little piece?

If you want the rationale on doing the smallest possible thing you can in the service of a much bigger goal, check out B. J. Fogg's work on tiny habits. And if you decided to do *nothing* on this exercise, or if you told yourself you'd come back and do it later, please just notice that tendency and consider whether it is part of a pattern that might be holding you back elsewhere. Then read on for a few more simple but powerful things you can do, try, and experiment with when you are feeling ready. These include some refreshing new options for eating, moving, commuting, and ... going to the bathroom.

Ditch Your Diet

One interesting thing to experiment with as you go about embracing Healthy Deviance is simply letting go of some of the things you've felt you *had* to do in order to be healthy. Dieting is one of those things.

Look, we can debate the merits of this or that diet. We can argue about study results. But it's important to remember that self-reported dietary data (the kind employed by most diet researchers) is notoriously unreliable. And studies done in clinical labs often have little to do with real-world conditions. All of that makes the large-scale, accurate tracking of what works and doesn't work in the realm of diet and nutrition close to impossible.

Mostly what the scientific literature shows is that the way people eat when they go on any kind of diet tends to rapidly regress into a form of eating quite similar to how they were eating *before* they went on that diet. As a result, many researchers have to come to the conclusion that most diets work about as well as most other diets.

This is not necessarily so (there's strong evidence that fat-free diets, for example, are particularly disastrous). But what's clear is that out in the wild of the real world, no diet works very well for very long. In fact, a comprehensive review of long-term dietary data conducted by a research team at UCLA suggests that *all* restrictive diets eventually fail and/or backfire, often leading subjects to gain back the weight they have lost, and then some.[37]

This has led the lead author of that review, Traci Mann, PhD, to conclude that most people would be far better off avoiding diets entirely. For more on that, see Mann's book *Secrets from the Eating Lab: The Science of Weight Loss, the Myth of Willpower, and Why You Should Never Diet Again.*

Interestingly, what *does* seem to work for most people over the long haul is by far the least tested, least restrictive, and least commercially hyped of all dietary approaches. It is not a diet at all. It's simply eating mostly real, whole, nutrient-dense foods and avoiding crappy, processed, addictive, inflammatory food-like products high in flours, sugars, oils, salt, and toxic additives.

There is some exciting new science to support this.[38] Consider this research, as reported by the *New York Times* in February of 2018:

> *Anyone who has ever been on a diet knows that the standard prescription for weight loss is to reduce the amount of calories you consume.*
>
> *But a new study, published Tuesday in JAMA, may turn that advice on its head. It found that people who cut back on added sugar, refined grains and highly processed foods while concentrating on eating plenty of vegetables and whole foods—without worrying about counting calories or limiting portion sizes—lost significant amounts of weight over the course of a year.*
>
> *The strategy worked for people whether they followed diets that were mostly low in fat or mostly low in carbohydrates. And their success did not appear to be influenced by their genetics or their insulin-response to carbohydrates, a finding that casts doubt on the increasingly popular idea that different diets should be recommended to people based on their DNA makeup or on their tolerance for carbs or fat.*
>
> *The research lends strong support to the notion that diet quality, not quantity, is what helps people lose and manage their weight most easily in the long run. It also suggests that health authorities should shift away from telling the public to obsess over calories and instead encourage Americans to avoid processed foods that are made with refined starches and added sugar, like bagels, white bread, refined flour and sugary snacks and beverages, said Dr. Dariush Mozaffarian, a cardiologist and dean of the Friedman School of Nutrition Science and Policy at Tufts University.*
>
> *"This is the road map to reducing the obesity epidemic in the United States," said Dr. Mozaffarian, who was not involved in the new study. "It's time for U.S. and other national policies to stop focusing on calories and calorie counting."*

Bless you, Dr. Mozaffarian. Blessings, too, to Dr. David Ludwig (a professor in the nutrition department at Harvard Medical School, and author of the terrific book *Always Hungry*) and to so many others who have tried to send this same message for many, many years now. Sadly, our country's nutritional dogma and policies have so far changed very little as a result of the study referenced above. The counsel of most doctors and registered dietitians, and the advice in most popular health and fitness magazines, remains shockingly focused on calories. It will probably take decades more for these findings to take hold in any way that is highly visible to the health-seeking public.

Why is this?

Because most experts have been brainwashed and peer-pressured into calorie-centric thinking. And because diets sell, and because processed foods (including diet foods) are hugely profitable. And because focusing on food quality versus quantity runs entirely counter to what all of us have been aggressively and repeatedly told to do for more than sixty years.

Just look at the way our Nutrition Facts Label is designed. Calories are in bold; carbs and fat grams are listed along with all sorts of other complex information that is largely useless and irrelevant but that demands our attention. The ingredient list, meanwhile, is small, innocuous, and often hard to find. We are not trained in how to interpret it, and we've not been trained to particularly care what it says.

Whole foods, meanwhile, have no ingredient labels at all. Raw meats and vegetables are intimidating to most people. We don't know how to deal with them. And, having eaten a lot of processed food, we simply don't find them nearly as palatable as the carefully architected combinations of sugar, flour, salt, fat, and flavorings that have been laboratory designed and tested to ensure that we cannot stop eating them.

The problem, of course, is that in a world that makes crappy, processed foods cheap, convenient, heavily advertised, seductively packaged, and biologically addictive, and that actively promotes diets as the way to be healthy and slender, choosing to eat mostly whole foods in a non-diet way is an unpopular, uncommon, and challenging thing to do—at least initially.

You know what makes it easier?

Not trying to do anything else.

Not counting calories. *Not* counting carbs, proteins, or fats. *Not* trying to eat specific quantities and ratios of things. *Not* trying to track every scrap you eat. *Not* trying to burn off every calorie you eat by spending a specific quantity of time going a specific speed at a specific elevation on a treadmill at the gym.

What makes it easier is just eating the whole foods that appeal to you and learning to choose, prepare, and combine them in ways that you genuinely enjoy. So, ditch your diet ...

Or Keep Your Diet

Look, if you can find a good, flexible, eating program that involves mostly whole foods most of the time and that leaves you feeling happy and satisfied and that also happens to be called a diet, far be it from me to tell you not to follow it. Do whatever works for you.

I've just found that most of the diet programs out there don't work well for much of anybody. And in all my years as a health journalist and a lifetime of my own experimentation, I've yet to find a single diet that shows any evidence of working better (over the short term *or* the long haul) than just eating mostly whole foods most of the time.

If embracing a whole-food approach to eating seems too aggressive for you right now, one smaller step could be simply steering clear of the most heavily processed foods in your midst. Again, I really don't want you to feel any pressure to adjust your eating while you are doing the Healthy Deviant Adventure program. But if you're feeling inclined to experiment with food-based alterations down the road, this is one relatively easy way to start.

According to a study of more than nine thousand people published in the medical journal *BMJ Open,* close to 60 percent of the food that American women, men, and children consume qualifies as "ultra-processed" foods, which the researchers defined as "formulations of several ingredients which, besides salt, sugar, oils, and fats, include food substances not used in culinary preparations, in particular, flavors, colors, sweeteners, emulsifiers and other additives used to imitate sensorial qualities of unprocessed or minimally processed foods and their culinary preparations or to disguise undesirable qualities of the final product."[39]

Pasta, for the record, despite commonly being made almost entirely from refined flours, was not included in that ultra-processed category. Americans eat a lot of pasta. Many American kids practically live on the stuff. And, as usual, all of this data was based on self-reported information pulled from the subject's twenty-four-hour dietary recall, not formal tracking. Plus, the study was based on 2009–2010 data. All of which means the actual percentage of ultra-processed foods in the U.S. diet today is probably *higher,* and the intake of actual, real, whole foods (meats, vegetables, eggs, nuts, seeds, unprocessed dairy) is probably quite a bit *lower.*

This report also found that 90 percent of the added sugar we eat comes from these ultra-processed foods. It notes that "foods higher in added sugars are often a source of empty calories with minimum essential nutrients or dietary fiber, which displace more nutrient-dense foods and lead, in turn, to simultaneously overfed and undernourished individuals."

This state of chronic, inflamed undernourishment is a big part of what is leaving us so depleted and vulnerable. It's also what's driving a huge amount of disease. According to that study, a high intake of added sugars increases the risk of "weight gain, excess body weight, and obesity; type 2 diabetes mellitus; higher serum triglycerides and high blood cholesterol; higher blood pressure and hypertension; stroke; coronary heart disease; cancer; and dental caries." Although not included in the above, Alzheimer's disease[40] has now also been tightly enough tied to blood sugar to have earned the nickname "type 3 diabetes."[41]

So if you value your body and mind, it seems clear that replacing even some of the ultra-processed foods you regularly eat with some appealing, nourishing real ones is one of the nicest, most Healthy Deviant things you can do for yourself.

Three Walks

Just as there is no prescribed diet in this book, there is also no prescribed exercise program. But for those of you who are now feeling the desire to move your body (a wonderful desire to heed), I offer you my Three Walks. They provide a fun, super-fast way to consciously reframe your experience of exercise and embrace movement as a conscious experiment in the body-mind connection.

I like to do one or more of the Three Walks (the "Slow Down," the "Straight Up," and the "Fast and Loose") whenever I am feeling down, tired, blah, irritated, or like the Unhealthy Default Reality is getting the better of me. I find that performing them shakes me out of my stupor, helping me reset mentally and emotionally while also energizing and recalibrating my body.

The Three Walks are also a nice thing to do first thing in the morning (as part of your Morning Minutes practice or after it is done) or during an Ultradian Rhythm Break. They are a superb thing to do after any meal; before a stressful meeting, conversation, or presentation; or whenever you feel like your body-mind could use a boost.

The goal of the Three Walks exercise is threefold:

- To put you into visceral contact with your body and let you unplug, momentarily, from the Unhealthy Default Reality

- To help you consciously notice what your body feels like in different and out of the ordinary sorts of motion, including unfamiliar postures, gaits, attitudes, and gestures

- To remind you what it feels like to move under your own steam while keeping your attention on your own experience versus some external self-fixing or self-betterment goal

I want to emphasize this point. The goal of the Three Walks is not to get you to exercise. The goal is not to get your heart rate up, to burn calories, to build lean muscle, or to tone or reshape any particular part of your body. Still, you will undoubtedly notice a different physical response to the unique (and in some ways surprising) challenges of each walk. You will likely also notice that the result of even a total of three minutes of these Three Walks has a remarkable impact on your body and mind.

Before you start walking, I'm going to suggest two quick preparatory steps:

First, pick a good place. You want a space that is large enough that you can walk around freely without bumping into furniture. A bigger room or back yard is ideal, but a greenway, park, track, golf course, playground, or any open, public space is also fine—as long as you don't mind people looking at you funny. If you *do* mind people looking at you funny, you are experiencing a classic obstacle to Healthy Deviance. This is how the Unhealthy Default Reality keeps you from doing all sorts of things you might otherwise do to take care of yourself. See how that works?

Next, decide how long you will do each walk. I recommend a minimum of one minute for each one. But you can also define your walks in terms of distance (for example, you could decide that you will walk from here to the other side of the room, to the mailbox, or around the block). Initially, plan to walk the same distance or time for each of the following Three Walks, just to get a sense of how they compare. Okay, that's it, here we go.

THE "SLOW DOWN" WALK

Walk in the way you usually do, but at approximately *half your normal pace*. To figure out what that pace is, first count off four steps as your feet hit the ground in your normal (likely rapid) walk: "1, 2, 3, 4." Next, take four steps at a pace timed to a count in which each foot remains on the ground for an extra count (most easily measured by counting "1 *and*, 2 *and*, 3 *and*, 4 *and*").

This will probably feel really odd, and you might notice that it is much more difficult to keep your balance when moving at this pace. That's because your brain is not currently programmed to walk this way; it's programmed to have you move at the pace you usually do. This is a huge, important Healthy Deviant insight to take note of:

It is easiest to move the way you usually do, at the pace you usually do, because your body-mind is wired for that.

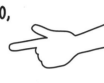

When you move your body differently or even envision moving differently, your brain begins creating new synaptic and proprioceptive networks to support that new reality. In the interim, what you get is weirdness. And that's okay. Just go with it for now.

Your mantra: *There is no rush. Slow is good. Be here now.*

- Notice how many more muscles are required in your lower legs and feet.
- Notice your core engaging as you wobble.
- Notice if you aren't sure how to move your arms when moving at this pace.
- Notice if you feel impatient to finish or like you are "wasting time."
- Observe your resistance to doing something differently than you usually do it.
- Get curious about what is going on in your body-mind as you take each step, and what it feels like to have to keep your attention on each step.

This is what *unfamiliar* feels like. It is not bad or good. It is just different. Practice tolerating this sort of difference, and you'll be building your Healthy Deviant neurology, musculature, and moxie all at once.

THE "STRAIGHT UP" WALK

Before you take any steps, draw yourself up to your full height, raise your chin, lift your chest, and drop your shoulders. Raise your vision toward a distant horizon. Take on the regal, dignified posture of a queen or king.

Now begin walking at a relatively slow, comfortable "processional" pace (the kind of pace you'd use walking down a wedding aisle or in a slow-moving parade). Keep your body relaxed, but poised and erect, as though you are wearing a crown and a cape, making the formal rounds, visiting this domain where you are the regal leader or sacred goddess of all you survey.

You might notice that it feels foolish to be walking in such a regal and dignified way. Nonetheless, continue to walk, taking graceful, thoughtful steps. Keep your body at full height, core engaged, your neck comfortably extended, your mind and your face calm, eyes soft, gaze elevated, jaw relaxed. As you walk, imagine looking around you with a placid, approving smile. All is well here in the realm. There is nothing pressing for you to do. Your time and attention are entirely your own to direct and enjoy as you see fit. Bask in that satisfaction as your complete your queenly or kingly walk.

Your mantra: *I am regal and dignified. I own and am pleased with all that I survey.*

- Notice whether taking a royal posture is challenging or easy for you, and whether it feels right or "put on."

- Notice any resistance you have to fully owning or taking responsibility for all that you survey (you cannot own people, obviously, and some might argue that you can't really own anything, but can you own their presence in your life at this time?).

- How does physically moving and holding yourself this way affect your mental and emotional state?

- How much attention and energy does it require not to maintain the habitual posture and pace you normally do?

- What would it be like, and how might people see you differently, if you were to assume a more dignified, self-possessed, regal posture during your normal life?

- In what ways might moving this way affect your attitude, choices, and behaviors?

THE "FAST AND LOOSE" WALK

Begin by shaking off all of the tension in your body. Wiggle and adjust your entire spine, hips, shoulders, and core. Wave and flop your arms and legs around, as though you are loosening up every joint in your body. Loosen up your jaw. Wiggle your fingers, toes. Tense and relax your face. Pull on your ears. Shake your head and hair out.

Next, take on the physical attitude of an energetic five-year-old. Look up at the sky and look all around you with wonder and delight. Begin walking like a happy, energetic little kid, flouncing and flopping, perhaps even hopping or skipping here and there.

Move at the most energetic pace you can muster, as though nothing is holding you back, but also as if you have nowhere in particular to go. You are in wild-and-free mode, loose on the world. Nobody is judging you. Nobody needs or expects anything of you. You are just having fun and enjoying the feeling of moving your body however it wants to move.

You might notice that it feels silly and embarrassing (but also kind of fun) to move so freely. Or you might notice that your body is tight and that it is hard for you to loosen up at all. Great. Exaggerate the swinging motions of your arms and legs. Allow your face to break into a childlike grin or a silly, goofy face. And continue covering as much ground as you can, walking or skipping as quickly as you comfortably can (without rushing), happily flopping with abandon as you go.

Put some vertical height into your movement, as though you have so much energy and joy in your child body that can barely contain it. Hold nothing back. Goofy grinning, giggling, snorting, singing, whistling, blushing, and gleefully saying "whee!" are all encouraged.

Take big breaths, inhaling and exhaling audibly. Get as much oxygen into your lungs as you possibly can, and also enjoy the feeling of breathlessness that comes as you exert yourself. Feel the blood rushing into your face and extremities.

Your mantra: *I'm free! Yay!*

- Notice how your body responds to moving in a way you might not have moved in years.

- How does physically moving and expressing like this affect your mental and emotional state?

- What does it feel like to inhabit the body posture of a much younger and perhaps substantially more energetic person?

- What would it be like for you to show the free, playful, happy side of yourself more often?

- Can you allow your body to move, your heart rate to rise, and your face to get flushed without feeling stressed?

WALKING YOUR OWN WAY

When I do the Three Walks exercise in workshops, the net effect is usually a group of pink-cheeked, shiny-eyed, happy-looking people who are energized, focused, standing straight, and excited to dive into the next session. I'm often amazed by how much more confident everybody appears. A number of participants have also noted this change and asked me if the Three Walks are based on Amy Cutty's power poses. They are not, but I suspect they elicit much the same neurologically mediated, empowering body-mind dynamics.

This is one of the things I love best about Healthy Deviant strategies. There are reams of good science that help explain why they work, but you don't have to be a scientist, understand the science, or even be aware of the science to make great use of them. For me, the best reason to do the Three Walks is to be reminded, viscerally, of some important Healthy Deviant truths, including the facts that:

- I am a free, autonomous, self-directed human being worthy of my own agency, attention, and care.

- I can choose my relationship to the world around me by going at my own pace and rhythm, and in directions of my own choosing.

- Moving my body through space feels good, and moving my body in unfamiliar ways, without the restrictions of having to "do it right," can feel great.

You might have a totally different response, of course, which is why I suggest trying these Three Walks for yourself and seeing what happens for you.

The Conscious Commute

The daily trips to and from work tend to be lost time for many people, and they also tend to be inherently stressful experiences that involve rushing, unpredictable traffic jams, missed trains or busses, and a general crush of humanity as everybody tries to get where they are going all at the same time.

One of my favorite ways to counter that dynamic, and to work micro-doses of Healthy Deviance into my days, is to practice conscious commuting. I consider it one of those small-scale revolutionary acts (or subtle jujitsu moves) that can have surprisingly big impacts. Conscious commuting is the practice of tuning in to your daily out-and-back experience and making it your own. It can involve:

- Allowing a few additional minutes for your trip with the goal of enjoying the drive, ride, or scenery (and potentially being able to stop if you encounter something fun or interesting along the way).

- Keeping your headspace quiet and calm rather than filling it with media, external noise, and other distractions.

- Seeing the drivers, passengers, pedestrians, cyclists, and other people you encounter along the way as fellow travelers rather than moving obstacles.

- Assuming an attitude of kindness, patience, and generosity, looking for opportunities to allow others to merge into your lane, or proactively waving them ahead of you in traffic rather than trying to beat them or block them out.

- Breathing deeply rather than holding your breath; relaxing your face, neck, and jaw rather than clenching them.

- Acknowledging, nodding politely, or making friendly eye contact with people you encounter rather than ignoring or scowling at them.

- Deciding you will get there when you get there rather than rushing and spending the entire commute awash in anxiety about being late.

- Actively choosing and practicing the mindset and mood you want to have when you arrive (at work or at home) while you are still en route to your location.

Obviously, you also need to be safe and use your own best judgment about when to smile at someone and about how you choose to engage with any given person you encounter, but one thing I noticed is that when I began actively managing my own mindset, started seeking connection with the people around me, rather than mentally distancing myself from them, I actually felt quite a bit safer. I also found myself feeling respect, affection, and communion (rather than apathy, prejudice, and fear) with a much broader spectrum of humanity. That often had an uplifting and inspiring influence on my days.

Even if you don't commute to work (maybe you work from home, or you're a stay-at-home parent, a caregiver, a student, or are institutionalized), consider how you might be able to actively adjust whatever transition time you typically have between the major parts of your days (even if that is a walk down the hall) in the service of your own health and happiness and in the service of showing up at your destination as the person you most want to be.

Go NOW

If there's one thing you can count on happening at least a few times a day, it's the need to go to the bathroom. For this reason, I see bathroom urges as a superb Healthy Deviant skill-building opportunity.

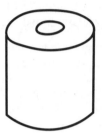

The Unhealthy Default Reality has convinced a lot of us that "holding it" is the right thing to do. We resist the urge to eliminate when we are too busy, too distracted, too mesmerized by the UDR to take stock of what really matters, or to show agency in our own self-preservation.

Here's the deal. Your body sends you the urge to pee or poop when it wants to excrete waste it no longer wants to carry around. When you insist on holding that waste inside your body, here's what you are doing:

- You're interfering with one of your body's most basic and essential functions.

- You're putting stress on important body parts (bladder, colon, urethra, and rectum).

- You're unnecessarily tolerating escalating levels of discomfort and distraction.

- You're retaining inflammatory toxic waste longer than you need to.

- You're giving that toxic waste an opportunity to be reabsorbed.

- You're setting the stage for constipation, urinary tract infections, and worse.

By ignoring the need to pee or poop when that need first makes itself known, you are, in effect, sending your body nasty messages like these:

- You don't matter much.

- I don't have time for you.

- Your needs can wait.

- I've got more important things to do.

- Your stress signals are just an annoyance to me.

- If you want me to hear you, you'll have to scream louder.

In the view of a Healthy Deviant, having to go to the bathroom is not an inconvenience; it is a privilege (ask anyone who has been catheterized or had to carry around a colostomy bag).

Any urge to go to the bathroom is also a tremendously important Amplified Awareness opportunity. Each and every act of noticing, stopping, and taking a trip to the bathroom teaches you the discipline of self-care. Each heeding of your body's need to eliminate waste affirms the sanctity of your body in a basic, nonnegotiable way.

Finally, going to the bathroom when you need to go—*at the moment you first need to go*—is also a profoundly important demonstration of autonomy. If you aren't willing to take care of your own bathroom needs, for goodness sake, where *are* you willing to advocate for yourself?

With this in mind, rather than ignoring the building pressure in your body, rather than waiting until you can't possibly wait another moment, or worse, waiting for the urge to recede (which definitely happens, with regrettable results), be on the lookout for that first subtle urge to go, and when it does, decide to *go now.*

Notice what interferes. That sense you should keep on working, that this is not a good time for a break, and that another time would be better. That feeling that your need to go to the bathroom may interrupt or inconvenience somebody else. That feeling that even acknowledging you have such bodily needs would be embarrassing.

Notice those socially programmed instincts to ignore your body, and then tell them to go to hell. Instead, when you *first* sense you've got any sort of waste matter headed for an exit, register that consciously, set aside whatever you are doing, politely excuse yourself (if necessary), and then proceed to the nearest bathroom and take care of your business. As you are doing that business, make a point of thanking your body for alerting you to its needs and for masterfully taking care of all the complex digestive and metabolic work it took to get things to this stage. Take a moment to reaffirm that you will be paying close attention to its future signals.

If you do this even a few times over the course of a single day, you will begin to notice that *this is what it feels like* to respect your body-mind and to heed its wisdom. You will begin wanting to do that in more ways, and more often.

Putting It All Together

Okay, so now you understand the power of Healthy Deviant perspectives. You get why breaking free of the Unhealthy Default Reality, even in small ways, is so essential to achieving, experiencing, and enjoying the things that matter most to you.

You also have a sense of how the Nonconformist Competencies, Renegade Rituals, and Healthy Deviant Survival Skills can help bust you loose from the Unhealthy Default Reality, allowing you to move beyond status-quo passivity, reactivity, and learned helplessness.

Now, it's time to learn from first-hand experience and experimentation how you can put all these things together in real-life practice and experience the power of Healthy Deviance for yourself.

In the chapters that follow, I walk you through a 14-Day Healthy Deviant Adventure program. This simple but radical two-phase approach to health reclamation integrates all three of the Nonconformist Competencies along with all three of the Renegade Rituals in the context of a fun, flexible program that will help you:

- Notice the ways in which you've been brainwashed and anesthetized into complicity with the Unhealthy Default Reality, and begin consciously reprogramming yourself for your own purposes.

- Make incremental adjustments in your daily choices based on real-time feedback.

- Restore your ability to regulate and direct your own energy and attention, and upgrade your ability to make sane, conscious, self-empowering decisions.

- Develop the basic skills you need to survive and thrive as a healthy person in our unhealthy society, and to help others to do the same.

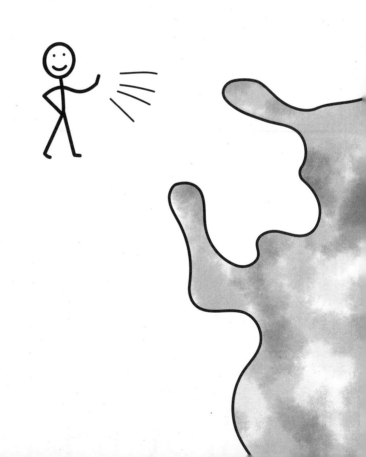

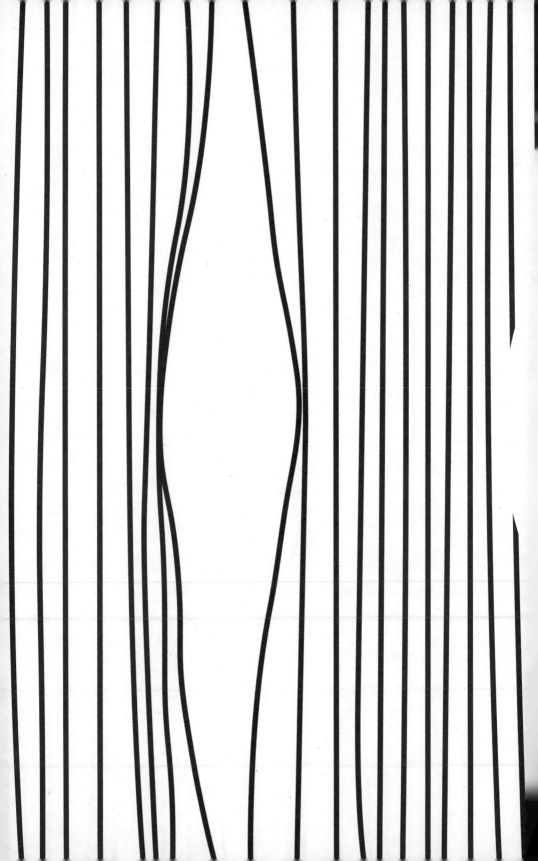

PART 4

Your Healthy Deviant Adventure

(A 14-Day Experiment in Radical Replenishment)

The greatest act of disobedience
in which you can engage is to begin to feel again,
to ask yourself every minute of every day, every time
you see something new in your field of vision:
HOW DOES IT FEEL?

—STEPHEN HARROD BUHNER

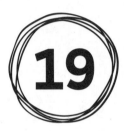

Get Ready for Weirdness

Life shrinks or expands
in proportion to one's courage.

—ANAÏS NIN

The minute you start messing with the Unhealthy Default Reality (UDR), things can and probably will start to get, um, weird. By that, I mean things will not be the way they have always been. You will not be the way you always have been. The life you've come to know and the person you think you are may both suddenly feel … different. Unfamiliar. Unpredictable. Odd. Quirky.

As you question your engrained assumptions and experiment with seemingly small changes to your established routines, your daily experiences will shift. Your "normal" patterns and reactions will begin to change—often in ways you don't initially understand or anticipate. Old structures might start to wobble. Long-binding restraints will start to loosen.

As you shift position and perspective, your visible horizon will open up and reveal new landscapes, new alternatives, and new ways forward. All of this may cause you to feel more free, energized, and hopeful. It may also cause you to feel a bit kooky and off-kilter. It's important to be prepared for this weirdness. It's also helpful to see it as the sign of progress it almost certainly is. Here's why:

Feeling unmoored is often the first sign that you have begun busting loose from the Unhealthy Default Reality.

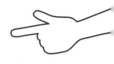

As you work through your Healthy Deviant Adventure, you may find yourself in an untethered relationship not just with the Unhealthy Default Reality, but with your own familiar habits, patterns, assumptions, and reactions. Even if you feel uncertain and a bit at sea, you may find yourself suddenly feeling a lot more clear headed and energized than you have in a long time. You may feel different in your body and mind—inclined to bounce more, breathe more, notice more, feel more. You may start flirting with new boundaries and experimenting with bold new choices.

As a result, you may find other people looking at you like, "Excuse me, but who *are* you?" You may start to feel like you aren't entirely sure how to answer that question.

That's all good. It means your Matrix-busting magic is working, and an exciting new phase of your Healthy Deviant journey has begun. But when our familiar, normal structures start to break down, even when those structures form the prison walls of a health-destroying dominant culture, it can feel strange and disconcerting.

Changing anything—even the automatic, default choices that have been keeping you stuck and suffering—almost always involves a moment of from-this-to-that transition. And at first, that moment can look and feel a lot like chaos. Old systems get disrupted. Cracks appear in your armor of normalcy. Questions begin to form around the edges of former certainty. The stale, warmed-over air you've been breathing is suddenly replaced by a fresh, cool breeze.

This can make you feel exposed, wobbly, and at risk. It can make you want to run for cover, abandon your experimental adventure, and retreat to the comfort of your old, familiar turf. Just for now, hang in there with me if you can. Stay on this ride a little longer, and I think you'll start to settle into a whole new groove.

How Healthy Change Really Happens

We are taught to believe that change happens like this: You decide to pursue a desired change, go for that goal, and make progress, and eventually—boom—the goal is achieved. Yay, you!

How often does it really work that way? Almost never. But that's the way all good before-and-after stories go, right? By the time our goals for healthy change are achieved, we are ready to forget about all the stuff we tried that *didn't* work, all the things we tried and failed, and instead just stick to the expected plot line. And so most of what we see and hear about healthy change makes it seem a lot simpler, easier, and more direct than it typically is.

Seen in its cleaned-up, camera-ready form, the path to healthy change looks like this:

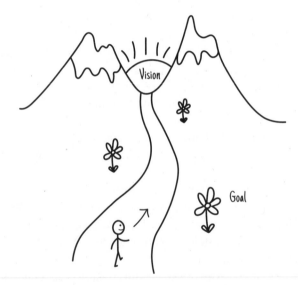

Seen from thirty thousand feet, it looks more or less like a straight-line trip. You start in one place, set yourself on a path to an inspiring vision, and accomplish a series of incremental goals on the way to your destination. Lovely.

But unretouched, seen up close and at human scale, that path may have dozens of switchbacks, temporary road closures, detours, construction zones, and confusing cloverleaf interchanges—moments when you're rerouted or thrown off track, or when you just plain lose momentum and find yourself back at a location that seems frustratingly close to where you started.

In reality, change more often works like this:

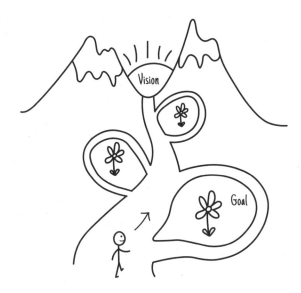

You think about a desired change for a while, perhaps a long while, and eventually, you decide it's worth pursuing. You may prepare or procrastinate for ages before you begin to take action. You may run into obstacles, run out of steam, or sink into the quicksand of your own unconscious resistance to change. You may surge forward with excitement, only to sink back into the grip of your oldest fear. You may take cautious steps, find yourself in uncharted territory, and run in the opposite direction of your stated goal.

When you get stuck in one of those seemingly infinite repeating loops or run into an unanticipated roadblock or find yourself suddenly heading up a steep, unmarked hill, it's easy to feel demotivated. It can feel like you're losing, like you're a failure, like you'll never reach your destination. You may berate yourself and convince yourself you are incapable or unworthy. You may decide this whole change thing is just not for you or not worth the bother. Until the pain or desire builds up again, and then ....

You will likely find yourself completing this advance-and-retreat pattern—from the familiar to the unfamiliar and back—many, many times over the course of any change effort. And perhaps many times during the course of a single day. That's totally okay. Those out-and-back experiences can be turned to your Healthy Deviant advantage (more on that in a moment). Just know the "weird" will come during your Healthy Deviant Adventure, and that it is a predictable part of escaping the UDR. Greet it with open-armed recognition and anticipation rather than trepidation and shutdown. Each time you do, it will seem more comfortable and less, well, weird.

Know that what you're experiencing is an essential discovery and growth process. It's a process of learning to see your path more clearly, identifying your patterns, assessing your relative areas of capacity and challenge. It's a process of developing the new wisdom and skills that will take you where you want to go. And guess what? Counter to what you may have been led to believe by a bunch of ridiculously truncated, oversimplified before-and-after makeover stories, *this is how it goes for everyone.*

In my fifteen years editing *Experience Life,* we received thousands of letters and success-story submissions from people who told us how they'd managed to profoundly change their bodies and their lives—often as the result of skills and knowledge they'd learned from the magazine. Never, not once, did I read the story of someone who had accomplished their healthy-change goals on the first go or learned everything they needed to know before they set out.

It just doesn't work that way.

So, here's the truth: No program—including this one—can completely spare you the experience of trying and faltering. What it *can* do is make the journey a much less halting and frustrating experience.

The goal of the Healthy Deviant Adventure is to give you a massive head start, spare you some avoidable detours and delays, get you through the messy parts with more dignity, empower you to arrive in better shape, and help you enjoy the trip. The program walks you down the road step by step and encourages you to regularly, repeatedly notice—without destructive reactions or judgments—just *where* and *how* you happen to meet with resistance, stumble, or temporarily forget that you're on a journey of your own choosing. Then it helps you shake off the dust, get reoriented, and hop right back on the path.

This program *assumes* you'll run into a certain amount of trouble. And really, that's the whole point. Noticing the mass-culture booby traps to which you are currently vulnerable, becoming aware of your own quirky patterns and trouble spots, learning to proactively reinforce yourself in ways that render you stronger and more resilient—these are the underpinnings of the Healthy Deviant Way. As you proceed along that way, you're developing the practices and perspectives that empower you to more regularly access the healthiest, happiest choices available to you. You're mastering the navigation tactics that get you past detours and pot-holed construction zones and onto a clearer, smoother, more direct path—a path, in short, that progressively begins to look and feel a bit more like that first picture.

As long as you keep identifying new visions, desires, and passions worth pursuing, there will *always* be new barricades and challenges cropping up on your path. Just think of them as new levels of game play—new opportunities to get smarter, stronger, and clearer. As with any complex video game, software program, or piece of music you decide to learn, the more engagement, willingness, and patience you bring to the challenge, the better you'll get at dealing with the tricky bits. The more challenge you can take on without getting frustrated and overwhelmed, the more you can accomplish—and create and give—with grace.

Being well prepared for weirdness (including potential surprises or trouble spots) is often a simple matter of having some sort of "if-then" plan. So, in the following brief sections, I'm going to give you a few pointers on what you can expect on your Healthy Deviant Adventure and what you can do to set yourself up for the best possible experience.

Big Picture Overview

Each of the two weeks in the Healthy Deviant Adventure program is designed to integrate daily thematic reflections with action-oriented experiments and energizing acts of self-care. But the two weeks also serve a somewhat different purpose:

- **Phase 1, "Start Where You Are,"** guides you to notice how even subtle changes to your daily mindset and habits can catapult you into a radically different relationship with the Unhealthy Default Reality. I want you to see that being gentle and compassionate with yourself can be more effective than being punishing, nitpicking, and slave driving.

- **Phase 2, "Raise Your Game,"** lets you leverage the newfound strength and awareness you unleashed in phase 1 by applying yourself with more intensity and rigor to the Healthy Deviant tasks at hand. This week is designed to bring you up against your resistance and triggers. It's designed to help you notice what happens when you start leaning a little harder against the often-invisible fences of the Unhealthy Default Reality—fences that are designed to keep you in.

How you use this two-phase program is up to you. You can complete phase 1 and then advance to phase 2, or you can move back and forth between phase 1 and phase 2, depending on how much energy you have on a given day. You can also repeat phase 1 for several months, experimenting with variations and combinations until you feel ready to move on to phase 2 *or* feel called to do something else entirely (like a Healthy Deviant program of your own making!).

What Each Day Holds

Each day of the 14-Day Healthy Deviant Adventure includes a consistent set of foundational components, including:

- A daily thematic Healthy Deviant reading (you might think of these as deviant devotionals).

- A series of Renegade Rituals (you get to choose which and how many you want to practice on any given day).

- Daily Deviance Journal Pages (fill them out as a way of experiencing your adventure more deeply, capturing field notes from your experiments, tuning into your present condition, and seeing your evolving experience play out on paper).

- Healthy Deviant Adventure Trackers (use them to chart your journey day by day and to notice shifting patterns in your vitality over time).

You can do these things at whatever times work for you at any point during the day, including *during* your Renegade Rituals. None of these activities requires huge effort or significant disruptions of your normal schedule. However, they will involve choices and produce effects different from your business-as-usual version of "normal." That is the whole point. Taken together, this series of small, disruptive steps amounts to a giant leap in the direction of Healthy Deviant autonomy. And, as noted, the result will be some weirdness, particularly at first. But by now, I think you are ready for that.

Each day has a consistent rhythm and flow that looks something like this:

A Day in the Life of a Healthy Deviant

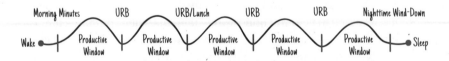

I encourage you to think about dividing your day into three primary parts and following a relatively consistent pattern if you can (feel free to adjust however you see fit based on your work schedule, special events, and so on). A given day might play out something like this:

MORNING

- Wake gently (no screens, no media, no stress)
- **Renegade Ritual: Morning Minutes**
- Conscious commute (or transition)

DAYTIME

- Arrival and preparation (at work or the site of your projects or pastimes)
- Productive window (an hour and a half to two hours of focused effort or attention)
- **Renegade Ritual: Ultradian Rhythm Break**
- Productive window
- Renegade Ritual: Ultradian Rhythm Break (you can incorporate lunch, *if* taken away from work)
- Productive window
- **Renegade Ritual: Ultradian Rhythm Break**
- Productive window
- Close up shop (save in-progress work; stack or file the random stuff in your work area, clean up any used glasses or coffee cups, jot down key to-dos for tomorrow, and so forth)
- Conscious commute (or transition)

EVENING

- Homecoming, reentry, dinner, evening activities
- **Renegade Ritual: Nighttime Wind-Down Ritual**
- Sleep

Whew! Okay, look, I know that at first glance that might look like a whole lot of things to do, but keep in mind that most of these activities (waking, going to work or school, doing your thing, coming home, eating, going to bed) are actions *you're already doing.*

Most of the Renegade Rituals can be accomplished within just a few minutes, and as a rule, they free up more time, energy, and effort than they consume, creating a net gain, not drain, on your resources. You'll find that they give you a level of clarity and equanimity that make other healthy choices seem more doable, more appealing, and more automatic over time.

The *best* thing about the Renegade Rituals is that they encourage you to briefly check in with yourself at regular intervals throughout the day, notice how you are doing, and reestablish your intentions to take good care of your Healthy Deviant self.

So actually, let's give those check-ins some visibility into your daily plan:

A Day in the Life of a Healthy Deviant

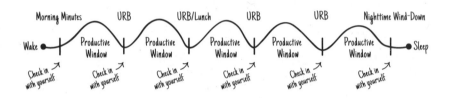

By establishing (really, just consciously respecting) this rhythm, you are prompting yourself to take stock of your present condition and real-life environment in a way few people ever do. Several times a day, you are making a conscious decision about what you will or won't do at a given moment, then acting on that decision and moving on.

Each time you do this, and particularly when you track the results, you disrupt your own status quo. You briefly separate yourself from your entrainment with the Unhealthy Default Reality—and in that moment, you alter it and its grip on you, however slightly. Do that repeatedly, with increasing levels of conscious awareness and autonomy, and you win.

Each time you complete a Renegade Ritual, consider marking it off on your Daily Deviance Journal Pages (thumbnails shown on opposite page). You'll find photo-copyable mini-samples of these worksheets in chapter 22, and you can download full-size, printable versions as part of the Healthy Deviant Workbook, available for download at HealthyDeviant.com/toolkit.

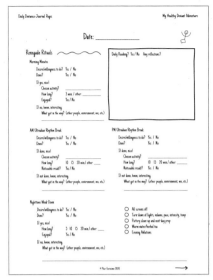

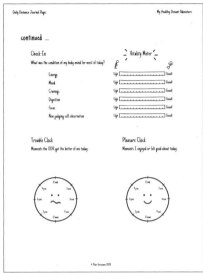

Before you go crazy with tracking your Renegade Rituals, though, or doing any part of the Healthy Deviant Adventure, I want to emphasize one more time for all you high-achievers out there: *You don't have to do every element of the program or do it perfectly for the program to work.* You just have to put your attention on what's happening, day by day, as you embrace, defer, or reject what's being offered—and as you begin to notice the patterns of your own response to the barriers that will inevitably arise.

The longer you do these things, the more natural and effortless and rewarding they will become. My hope is that you'll want to repeat some version of these Healthy Deviant reflections, actions, and practices for the rest of your life. But first, a few practical preparatory tasks …

Before You Go Rogue

Here are a few suggestions for setting up your space and schedule, gathering necessary goods, and enrolling social support.

CHOOSE YOUR SPOTS

Decide where you will do your Morning Minutes and at least some of your Ultradian Rhythm Breaks.

- Ideally, your chosen spots will be calm, quiet spaces where (for the period of at least a few minutes) you won't be interrupted or disturbed and where you can safely lower or turn off electric lighting and control sound.

- For those with multi-room homes or apartments or those who live alone, this might be a kitchen table or counter, dining room, living room, or den.

- If you have small children or live in a small space with roommates, your only option may be your bedroom, a bathroom, an alcove, a basement or attic, or some other improvised space (perhaps a square you mark on the floor with masking tape or a nook between a piece of furniture and the wall).

- Clear as much clutter as you can from the immediate vicinity and from your direct line of sight.

- Dust and wipe clean any dirty surfaces within touch or view (no need to be obsessive about it; just remove any evident filth with the intention of making the space ready for an intentional act of sacred self-care).

- Make sure you can safely burn a candle without damaging or lighting anything on fire.

- Do whatever else you can and want to do to make the space comfortable, attractive, free of clutter, and appealing to your senses (you might screen or move out any ugly junk or stress-triggering objects, create a small altar, have a favorite essential oil to waft around, or place some objects of beauty or significance nearby).

- Avoid launching into any major remodeling, painting, or redecorating projects that will delay your start (procrastinating perfect-preparers, you know who you are!).

- Aim to spend between ten minutes and an hour identifying and readying your chosen spaces.

ASSEMBLE YOUR TOOLS

You'll want to have the following available:

- A simple, pleasant-to-wake-to alarm clock or some wake-up tool that is not your cell phone, tablet, laptop, or other complex, wifi-connected device (see Step-by-Step Practice Tips for Morning Minutes in chapter 15 for some suggested options).

- Something to sit on (could be a chair, yoga mat, cushion, or folded blanket on the floor).

- A stable, clear surface, such as a table, counter, un-upholstered stool, bench, or bit of floor within easy reach.

- An unscented candle (get real beeswax if at all possible; choose votives or pillars over tippy, fast-burning tapers).

- Some matches or a lighter.

- A small dish or other smooth, heat-safe surface to place the candle on and to catch any melted wax.

- A simple timer that allows you to set a three-minute or longer alarm (again, ideally this would *not* be your cell phone, but if that's all you've got, it'll work).

- This book or a hard copy of this book's program pages for the current day (printable downloads available at HealthyDeviant.com/toolkit).

ANNOUNCE YOUR INTENTIONS

Start by announcing your Healthy Deviant Adventure plans to yourself. Next, consider telling the people you live with that you are doing some new practices as an experiment, and you'd be grateful for their support.

- Don't feel obliged to explain anything else about your Renegade Rituals unless you are feeling a strong desire to do so.

- If announcing that you're embarking on a Healthy Deviant Adventure is likely to raise more eyebrows than you care to, consider framing it as a "science-based health-improvement program" or "a series of exercises for improving energy and focus" (which it is).

- Know that this may be your first act of Healthy Deviant boundary setting. Expect resistance, ridicule, and even potential sabotage.

- If you don't like the idea of telling anybody about your plan, and think you'll get less resistance by doing it without any announcement or fanfare, follow that instinct.

- You may or may not have to tell anybody at work about your plan to take Ultradian Rhythm Breaks. If you have a regular desk job and are subtle about it, you probably aren't going to be missed. If necessary, you could potentially take a URB without even leaving your workspace. If you work on a factory assembly line or some other tightly regulated job, you may need to take these breaks at assigned times or grab them as "bathroom breaks" (in which case, you'll probably have to keep them significantly shorter than twenty minutes).

- Make sure you know your rights. While OSHA regulations are woefully remiss in not mandating or providing paid breaks, many states have stricter requirements. Most decent employers provide for breaks or are open to negotiating around them for health and safety reasons. If you need to, seek counsel and support from a workers' rights advocacy group.

- Consider making a business case for your breaks. Your employer may be open to looking at some of the scientific literature on ultradian performance rhythms, or relevant industry research on breaks and productivity in general. One great resource to suggest to any efficiency- and performance-oriented manager is a classic 2003 book on training "corporate athletes," *The Power of Full Engagement: Managing Energy, Not Time, Is the Key to High Performance and Personal Renewal* by Jim Loehr and Tony Schwartz.

- Above all, keep in mind that by taking regular URBs, you are doing your employer's business *a favor.*

PREVIEW AND MARK YOUR CALENDAR

You can do the Healthy Deviant Adventure whenever you like, but if you work a regular Monday-to-Friday job, it might be easiest to do your prep work over a weekend and begin the program on a Monday.

- Take a look at your upcoming schedule and see if there are any deal-breakers within your planned Healthy Deviant Adventure time horizon.

- Keep in mind that busy, stressful times can actually be the *best* times to do this program.

- Initially, mark only the seven days of phase 1 on your calendar (on the final day of phase 1, you'll be deciding whether to repeat phase 1 or move onto phase 2).

- If you use a digital calendar, add an all-day event that spans all included days; if you use a paper calendar, mark or highlight those days however you see fit.

POST SOME REMINDERS

Because you are going to be challenging a lot of automatic, pre-programmed, default behaviors, it can help to have visual triggers that remind you of what you are doing different from normal and why.

- Consider strategically placing one or more of pieces of Healthy Deviant signage (located in the Healthy Deviant Toolkit) around your space as environmental prompts.

- Supplied signs include a day-by-day check-off list, tent cards, and hang tags in a range of sizes ideal for posting on your mirror, fridge, desk, car dashboard, and other locations. Feel free to customize them or make your own from scratch, and put them wherever you like.

- Consider moving the signs around, even on the surface of the same location, from day to day. This reduces the likelihood of your ceasing to see them and increases their useful lifespan.

DO SOME WARM-UP EXERCISES

If you aren't feeling quite ready to dive into the Healthy Deviant Adventure, the following optional interactive and reflective exercises can function like deep knee bends for the body-mind, helping you get centered, focused, and motivated to take your next steps:

- **Your Ideal Day Visualization:** This guided visioning and meditation session by yours truly (available as a free MP3 at HealthyDeviant.com /toolkit) helps you summon the clarity, courage, and motivation to see your best self with fresh eyes, and to pursue your chosen daily reality with new energy.

- **Healthy Deviant Hero's Journey Mapping:** Read part 2 of this book ("The Making of a Healthy Deviant") and circle your current position within the Healthy Deviant Hero's Journey. Note where you are likely headed next.

- **Your Trouble Clock:** This illuminating review of your own daily patterns (see below) helps reveal where you're currently most vulnerable to temptation and self-sabotage. It also offers some insights into why that might be so, and suggests how to use your own weaknesses to your advantage.

Reading Your Trouble Clock

We all have them—our weird little moments of unconsciousness, apparent weakness, and strife. Those times when we feel triggered or vulnerable to making unconscious and less-than-healthy choices. Those times we later regard with regret, frustration, or vague bewilderment—as in, "Ack, why did I do *that* again?"

Although those moments may seem to just happen, they typically occur (and recur) at the same places and within the same windows of time—often times when we are lonely, bored, stressed, hungry, or otherwise physically or emotionally depleted. The bulk of the rest of our hours don't seem to pose as much of a problem, likely because we are:

- Running "on automatic" in the flow of demands that don't allow us much room to waver.

- In relatively conscious command of our choices.

- Being observed by others.

- Sleeping.

Placed against this background of business as usual, our contrasting unhealthy patterns tend to stand out like sore thumbs. And, like sore thumbs, they don't come out of nowhere. On the contrary, they are typically the symptom of some injury or insult that preceded them.

With this in mind, rather than seeing our unhealthy patterns as random aberrations (and feeling victimized by them when they occur), it can help to simply visualize them on a twenty-four-hour Trouble Clock. When you do, you may notice that they are surprisingly predictable and reliable occurrences—moments often preceded by (or immediately preceding) periods of imbalance, over-exertion, stress, disconnection, and lack of essential inputs.

In my own life, I've found that most of my Trouble Clock patterns can be explained by what happened in the two hours prior to the trouble. Breaks and meals I missed. Stress I endured. Problematic foods or drinks I consumed. Toxic exchanges I tolerated. Healthy pleasures I denied myself.

Looking at your Trouble Clock provides you with an illuminating review of where you're currently most vulnerable to temptation and self-sabotage. It may also give you some insights into why that might be so. Many filled-in Trouble Clocks reveal that periods of craving, reduced energy, temptation, and emotional reactivity are reliably preceded by periods of extended stress, or by a high output of energy (big meeting, big project, big workout) followed by inadequate recovery or replenishment.

Observing our own moments of perceived "weakness" in this way can help us gain a distinct advantage over them. It gives us the opportunity to appreciate the powerful role that our conditions and current state play in creating our vulnerabilities (cravings, fatigue, emotional reactivity) of the moment. It can also help us begin consciously preparing for and responding to our personal moments of challenge in ways that serve us better. A blank Trouble Clock might look something like this:

Trouble Clock

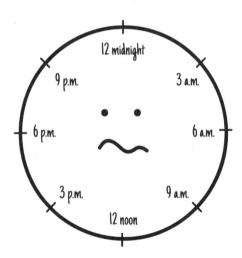

Throughout the day and evening, there are a great many places we might encounter temptation, compulsion, depletion, reactionary choices, and other forms of what I call "Trouble" with a capital T. If you close your eyes for a moment and try to conjure up a few Trouble spots of your own, I bet you can picture them. You are doing a thing you know doesn't serve you, a thing you wish you didn't do (or do quite as much), maybe a thing you wouldn't want others to know about or witness, a thing that costs you and causes you to suffer.

As noted, I find that periods of Trouble are reliably preceded by periods of excess stress or by depletion that occurred in the previous two hours or so. For me, this often looks like some a protracted or extreme output of energy or endurance, followed by inadequate recovery or replenishment. Classic culprits include stress, anxiety, refined carbohydrates, alcohol, dehydration, and having gone too long without a break.

Once populated, a Trouble Clock might look like this:

Filled Trouble Clock

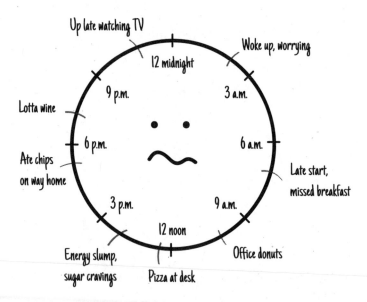

Right now, take a moment to mentally walk through an ordinary day, and on a blank piece of paper or on the Trouble Clock portion of a Daily Deviance Journal Page (see Healthy Deviance Toolkit, chapter 22), mark down a few moments you identify as "trouble spots" of your own.

Don't feel you have to mark *every* instance of Trouble; just focus on those that occur with the greatest regularity and that cause you the most consternation. If it's an experience or event that often leaves you feeling lousy, frustrated, frayed, tempted, unconscious, numb, or regretful, mark it down. Then notice the following:

- What was going on in the two or so hours preceding your Trouble?

- What was your stress level like leading up to Trouble?

- When, prior to Trouble, did you last have a break, hydration, or good, nutrition-dense, whole-food nourishment (as opposed to caffeine, sugar, flour, fast food, junk food, and so on)?

- When was the last time you got to experience some pleasure, relaxation, self-care, social support, or fun?

Filling in Your Trouble Clock

Following are just a few examples of common Trouble patterns. But I'm sure you'll have your own original contributions to make. And as you embark on the Healthy Deviant Adventure, you'll inevitably discover more. For now, as you review the list, just mark any that sound familiar, and jot down any similar or corollary tendencies you're aware of in your own life.

EARLY MORNING

- You get up and feel tired, so you skip your workout.

- You're not hungry, so you skip breakfast.

- All you feel like eating is toast—maybe a lot of toast.

- You skip taking your vitamins or meds because it's too much trouble or you don't have time.

- You can't find your keys, wallet, phone, purse, or files, and looking for them causes you to be late, rushed, and frantic.

- You leave the house without a water bottle or healthy snack for later.

- You can't resist grabbing a pastry at the bakery down the street.

- You overdo it on coffee or sugar and wind up feeling rattled and wired.

- You arrive late to work and have to rush to a meeting or dive headlong into a project without getting settled first.

MIDMORNING AND MIDAFTERNOON

- You are tempted by donuts, cookies, cake, or other supplied goodies in the break room.
- You get hungry, so you hit the vending machine or convenience store across the street.
- You meant to bring a lunch but didn't, so you get fast food or pizza or eat whatever is available (like cold cereal, instant oatmeal, or baby carrots).
- You feel hungry or want to nibble on something shortly after eating.
- You hit the coffee shop for chai, frappe, mocha, caramel latte, or some other sweet thing and pick up some pastry or candy while you're there.
- You drink soda or sweetened coffee drinks at your desk or cruise by the office candy jar several times a day.
- You forget to drink water.
- You are too busy to go to the bathroom.
- You sit motionless at your desk for long periods of time, even when your back and neck start to hurt.
- You feel fatigued or distracted, perhaps on the verge of falling asleep.

COMMUTE HOME

- You nibble or drink sweetened drinks while you drive.
- You grab groceries on the way home and grab a little something sweet or salty to eat while you shop.
- You grab a bag of snacks to eat in the car.
- You skip a planned workout because you're pressed for time, the gym parking lot looks full, or you don't have the energy.
- You opt out of yoga, because you just aren't feeling it or forgot your yoga clothes or mat.
- You meet friends for happy hour on the way home and wind up having more drinks and chicken wings or jalapeno poppers than you planned.

BEFORE DINNER

- You're inclined to have one or more cocktails or glasses of wine to relax, or you smoke pot, which leaves you open to other temptations.

- You have crackers and cheese on tap the whole time you are preparing the evening meal.

- You still have a lot of work to do, so you set up your computer or get on the phone and keep working.

- You can't face any more work so you do some "unwinding" in front of the television, computer, or game console.

- You don't interact much with your partner or other members of your household because your head is still full of work thoughts, you're feeling prickly or stressed out, or you're too busy "unwinding."

- You realize you don't have groceries or don't feel like cooking, so you go out, order food delivered, heat up a frozen pizza, pop something questionable in the microwave, or figure you'll just skip dinner and cobble together some snacks from what you have on hand.

DINNER

- You settle for food you know isn't good for you and that may not even appeal to you.

- You put more food on your plate than makes sense because you don't want to deal with leftovers.

- You eat standing at the counter, over the sink or garbage can, or from a pan, disposable container, or dish.

- You load up on refined carbs (pasta, bread, pizza crust, rice, or couscous).

- You don't eat many (or any) non-starchy veggies, either because you don't have any on hand, you don't know how to prepare them, you don't like them, or they just don't seem appealing right now.

- You take multiple servings of less-healthy foods that you just can't seem to get enough of.

- You aren't hungry, or you feel like you ate too much during the day, so you don't eat much or you make some popcorn or another snack to enjoy while you watch television.

AFTER DINNER

- You forget to take (or just don't feel like taking) your evening vitamins, minerals, supplements, or medications.

- You binge-watch television shows or movies.

- You turn on news, which makes you sad, mad, scared, or depressed.

- You snack in front of the television or repeatedly go to the kitchen to nibble.

- You eat ice cream from the carton—maybe the whole carton.

- You get sucked into social media, video games, or other electronic pastimes.

- You have one or multiple alcoholic drinks or sweetened beverages.

- Not long after eating, you feel bad about overeating—or you realize that you're still hungry and are compelled to eat more.

- You avoid doing work or projects you'd planned to do because you are too worn out or just don't feel like it.

- You have conflicts or feelings of separation with the people you live with.

- You spend a lot of the time on the phone with a friend or family member who always seems to need counseling or wants to commiserate, leaving you with little time for yourself and the people you live with.

- You feel anxious, sad, or lonely unless you are occupied with a distraction or something to do.

- You do some online shopping or peruse catalogs even though there's nothing in particular you need.

- You find a reason to leave the house, because you don't like being there.

BEDTIME

- You feel like you have too much to do, so you stay up too late working or doing chores.

- You feel like you just need to tune out, so you watch television or movies for an hour (or two or three).

- You have an alcoholic drink (or two or three) before you retire to help you wind down.

- You fall asleep on the couch or in front of the television.

- You roll into bed without having washed your face and brushed and flossed your teeth.

- You are hungry for a bedtime snack but struggle with what to eat or whether you should eat anything at all.

- You are hungry for a bedtime snack, so you open a bag of snacks or clean up all the leftovers.

- You feel lonely or bored or in need of stimulation, so you turn to porn, which leaves you feeling weird, frustrated, ashamed, or some other way you don't like feeling.

- You are turned on and feel like making love with your partner or sensually enjoying yourself, but you don't (for whatever reason), and then you can't sleep because you're sexually worked up or frustrated.

- You are worrying and thinking about things and can't get to sleep, so you toss and turn or just lie there with your brain working overtime.

MIDDLE OF THE NIGHT TO EARLY MORNING

- You wake up—worried, thinking, hungry, sweating, cold, lonely, or all of the above—and can't get back to sleep.

- You are woken by a baby, pet, partner, or family member who can't sleep or needs help.

- You go stand in front of the fridge and decide to have a midnight snack.

- You eat something you denied yourself at dinner or didn't want to eat in front of other people.

- Since you're awake anyway, you decide to get some more work done or watch late-night television or mess around on the computer.

- You finally fall asleep only to be woken by your alarm, which feels like it is going off way too early.

Your Pleasure Clock

You'll note that your Daily Deviance Journal Pages include a counterpart to your daily Trouble Clock—namely, your daily Pleasure Clock. I included this tool as a way of encouraging you to reflect on the parts of your day you find delightful, rewarding, satisfying, or just noticeably nicer than the rest of your day.

Marking these moments down and taking time to reflect on them amounts to savoring, and savoring experiences allows you to reexperience and magnify their benefits.

Your ability to savor positive experiences is correlated with—and may help determine—your level of mental health.[42] Some studies are exploring the power of savoring to offset chronic pain and even to treat opioid addiction.[43]

Biochemically speaking, anticipating, savoring, and

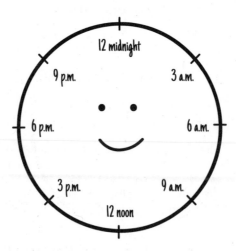

Pleasure Clock

reflecting on the best parts of your day all help amplify your body's release of feel-good neurochemicals, peptides, and ligands. It also helps your brain to lay down bigger and better neural networks for noticing and processing pleasure, which, in turn, predisposes you to creating more of those moments and to taking more pleasure in them in the future.

I'm a big believer in the adage "what you put your attention on grows" (and this notion is supported by reams of neuroscience demonstrating how mental focus affects perception). While paying close attention to what gives you trouble can be illuminating and informative, paying attention to your pleasure, noticing the parts of your life that are working well, can be even more rewarding in the long run. Consider how you might be able to use deliberate infusions of healthy pleasure as a way of warding off Trouble.

Filled Pleasure Clock

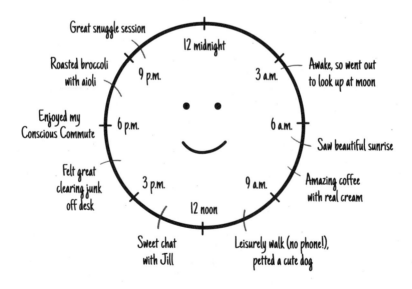

Unraveling an Obstacle

Whenever you find that you are doing something you want to *stop* doing, but can't, or when you find that you want to *start* doing something, but do not, you have a prime Healthy Deviant opportunity on your hands.

Use your Core Competencies to unpack and rethink it.

- First use Amplified Awareness to notice precisely how and when it occurs, or what gets in the way of it occurring (Trouble Clock).

- Next, use Preemptive Repair to get ahead of the depletion, overwhelm, or interference that is precipitating it (Renegade Rituals).

- Finally, use Continuous Growth and Learning to study and experiment your way to creative solutions, interventions, and alternatives that work for you.

As you encounter and meet your obstacles with these new tools and methods, you will find they start to undo themselves in ways that surprise you. Okay, all set? Let the Healthy Deviant Adventuring begin.

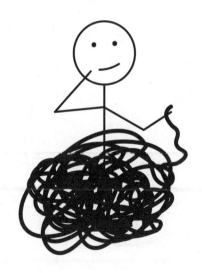

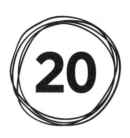

PHASE 1

Start Where You Are

Start where you are. Use what you have.
Do what you can.
—ARTHUR ASHE

DAY 1

Wake Up

Let the things that enter your life wake you up.
—PEMA CHÖDRÖN

Welcome. Today is an experiment in regaining (and retaining) consciousness.

Waking up is the first step. Not just waking up from sleep (although that is necessary). It's more about waking up from the hypnotizing, miasmic, life-force depleting coma that is the Unhealthy Default Reality. Waking from the spell of the Unhealthy Default Reality (UDR) involves nudging, tapping, singing, and shaking awake the powerful, wise, and autonomous parts of yourself that are present, but semi-dormant.

Waking up is comparatively easy. Staying awake is the tough part. Because waking up and finding yourself in the UDR is not always pleasant. In fact, it can be profoundly disorienting. That's just how the UDR rolls.

The UDR, remember, is a world where the unhealthy choices are easy and convenient, appealing, and affordable. It's a world where you are never good enough, where you have endless problems and advertisers have an endless array of products that promise to solve them, but somehow never do. Why? Because the problem isn't *you*. The problem is the UDR.

The UDR surrounds and mesmerizes you in a thousand different ways. It warps your vision. It dulls your senses. It drains your energy. It simultaneously numbs and frays your nerve endings. It robs you of opportunities to reflect, repair, and recover. And it has been doing that to you for a long, long time.

The UDR would very much like to keep you in a state of suspended animation. It would like to siphon off your resources, your clarity, your confidence, and your autonomy. Because the less strong, capable, clear headed, and self-directed you are, the easier you are to subdue, to draw in, to feed on, and to keep captive.

As noted, the UDR is, in effect, the crazy that passes for normal (see part 1 for more on that). And today, you will see that "normal" through fresh, clear eyes. You will see it in the pastries and candy and novelty treats that dominate checkout lines and invite impulse buys. In the energy drinks and soft drinks that are easier to find than clean, good-tasting tap water. In the caramel-almond-chocolate-toffee syrups and trans-fat-laden, artificially flavored nondairy creamers that come with coffee. In the fries and chips that are served with lunch. In supersized fast food and fun-sized everything. In two-for-one junk-food bargains. In supposedly healthy low-calorie, fat-free, zero-carb, cholesterol-free processed foods that are really just another form of trickily disguised junk food.

You'll see it in the fact that simple, whole, healthy foods are generally much harder to find and more expensive, less convenient, less enticing, and more time consuming to eat than everything else. You will see it in your too-long commute. You'll see it in your stressful, sedentary job—or in your rushed and physically exhausting job—and in the limited opportunities you have to move in ways that feel good or connect with people you enjoy.

You might even see it in the overly aggressive workout you're putting your body through because you think you have to, even though you keep getting injured, because it's the workout everybody else is doing. You'll see it in the recovery days you aren't observing because you don't dare stop.

You'll see it in the addictive allure of your smartphone and the thousand other screens that surround you, day and night, with irresistible distractions and impossible ideals. You'll see it in bikini-body magazine covers and the streaming, blaring, overstimulating media that is everywhere, always. You'll see it in the time you spend looking in the mirror, obsessing about your imperfections, judging yourself against impossible standards, and comparing yourself to all of the people you think are achieving those standards.

You'll see it in the temptation to buy something, anything, just this one thing, because you must have it now, and it's available now, for a limited time only, at a discount too good to pass up, and because it seems like it will make your life better—and besides, everybody else is getting one just like it. In the credit card bills that make your heart sink and your pulse race. In the temptation to stay up too late; to drink too much, smoke too much, vape too much, caffeinate too much, and watch too much TV; to get stuck in a social-media vortex or gaming vortex so powerful that you just can't pull yourself away, even when you're exhausted.

You'll see it in the gravity blankets and fidget spinners and anti-anxiety meds and supplements (CBD, anyone?) that you use to calm yourself down. You'll see it in all of the things that make your life feel slightly more bearable by allowing you to feel and notice less, the things that allow you to wrap yourself in a comforting cloak of numbness—even though you know, at a deep level, that that cloak is working against you. Because it is allowing you to endure the unendurable.

Over time, enduring the unendurable breaks you down. Enduring the unendurable is exactly what the UDR wants you to do. So today is the wake-up day. Today is the day you open your eyes to all of this, and you begin seeing the world, and your place in it, differently.

You are awake now. Look around, see the UDR for what it is. Feel yourself for who you are, and tap into the inherent dignity and humanity of your personhood, separate from the UDR. See how long you can hang onto your conscious awareness and autonomy before the UDR lulls you back into complacency.

Can you last fifteen minutes? An hour? Two hours? Keep watch, and keep track. The Renegade Rituals will help.

- Use the Morning Minutes to amplify your awareness and connect with your newly awake self.

- Use your Ultradian Rhythm Breaks to preemptively repair, detoxify, reorganize, and reinforce yourself before you become vulnerable and reactive.

- Use your Nighttime Wind-Down to disconnect from the outside world and prepare for a deeply restful, healing sleep—one that equips you to wake up stronger and clearer than the day before.

Then wake up again. For real. Keep doing that.

Remember: Here's how it used to be.

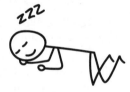

Here's how it is today.

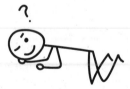

This is a good place to start.

Check in with your newly awakened self and ask: "Are you willing to do one or more Renegade Rituals today?" Put those rituals in your schedule. Set reminders and alerts. Otherwise, you might be surprised how quickly the UDR reaches out to grab you with its tentacles and rock you back asleep.

DAY 2

Gather Courage

Not everything that is faced can be changed,
but nothing can be changed until it is faced.

—JAMES BALDWIN

Welcome back. How did yesterday go? Here are some likely possibilities:

- Um, I can't remember. (A sign the Unhealthy Default Reality [UDR] got to you and sucked you back in—totally normal, and good to notice!)

- Kind of weird. I suddenly started seeing how many ways the UDR is operating in my life, and frankly, it freaked me out. (Also totally normal, and good to notice!)

- I am not sure. I don't know what to think. I'm still trying to decide how I feel about all of this. (Also totally normal, and good to notice!)

- Holy crap, the way I've been living is crazy, it has been killing me, and I need to change it. (Totally normal, and good to notice!)

- Some combination of the above, or something else entirely:

_____

(Also totally normal, and good to notice!)

The point of yesterday was to become newly conscious of your current relationship to the UDR, and then notice what it is like to consciously alter that relationship, even subtly, by virtue of your Amplified Awareness of it.

Initially, this just involves being awake enough to notice (even with one eye barely peeping open) that the UDR is there and that you are in relationship with it. But this "just noticing" is no small thing. In fact, it is huge, because most people aren't noticing, and that is what gives the UDR its power.

After the noticing comes the seeing. Then (as you are able to stay awake longer) there will likely be a series of coming-to-grips moments—a progressive reckoning with what *is*, with how the UDR has been really affecting you, and what you will now choose to do about it.

All of this can be intense, discombobulating, and potentially overwhelming. So today, we gather courage. We summon those resources that are innate and inviolable within us and that remain forever beyond the reach of the UDR. We reclaim our right to wield these precious, powerful resources on our own behalf.

Courage is one of those resources. Acceptance is another. Willingness is a third. We'll be covering acceptance and willingness on days 3 and 4. So for now, let us focus on courage.

Courage, in essence, is persisting and advancing in the face of fear. It is the decision (or, in some cases, the gut instinct) to feel the fear and do it anyway. Courage is not ignoring or denying your fear. Courage is deciding that you can be bigger than your fear, bigger than the real and imagined obstacles standing in your way.

One of the tricky things the UDR does, though, is make us feel small, weak, pathetic, cynical, uncertain, and incapable. It fractures our energy and attention, so we have a hard time accessing the central threads of love and courage that run within us. It places us in a hall of mirrors where our fears are multiplied and magnified, convincing us that they are far too much for us to overcome and that we need to focus on merely surviving, enduring, and getting by. That's how the UDR keeps us stuck.

When we choose to alter our relationship with the UDR, here are some of the most basic fears we face:

- Fear of trying, failing, and finding ourselves back where we started—or worse

- Fear of trying and succeeding—and then what?

- Fear of what others will think of us and how they will relate to us

- Fear that we will lose power or position or approval

- Fear that if we stop pushing so hard and running so fast we will get fat, get fired, become broke, boring, lazy, homeless, and so forth

- Fear that we are not worthy of this much special effort or attention

- Fear that letting go of our current structures and strictures (painful as they might be) will leave us without any foundation or identity at all

- Fear that (fill in the blank): _____

_____

_____

Look, change is just plain scary. Change in the face of an entire dominant culture that doesn't want you to change is even scarier. It requires courage (as well as energy and focus) we may not feel we can access, particularly in our depleted, UDR-captive state.

Want to gather your courage? Try using your fear as fuel. Notice where it sits in your body (your chest? your stomach? your neck? your knees?). Feel the fear vibrating and coursing through your body. Now imagine that it is not fear, but excitement, exhilaration, anticipation, raw energy, and potential. Ask yourself: "What if I used this powerful energy to change my life for the better?" Now imagine that energy pulsing, as pure courage, through all your veins, making you invincible.

Decide you will run some bold (yet safe) courage-stoking experiments today, starting with your Renegade Rituals. Don't allow the UDR to terrify, addle, distract, or anesthetize you into submission. Feel your fear and resistance about making even these small self-empowering changes, and then do them anyway. If you can't bring yourself to do even one Renegade Ritual, just *imagine* doing them. Pay attention to what happens. Use your Daily Deviance Journal Pages to record the results.

Okay, so what's your Renegade Ritual plan for today? Morning Minutes? Ultradian Rhythm Breaks? Nighttime Wind-Down?

Ha, Ha! Take *that,* UDR.

DAY 3

Find Things Right

When we stop opposing reality,
action becomes simple, fluid, kind, and fearless.
—BYRON KATIE

Yesterday we reflected on the importance of gathering courage to face the challenges of the Unhealthy Default Reality (UDR) and the creepy-crawly fears that often come to visit when we set out to extract ourselves from its clutches.

Today, we're going the other direction, exploring the power of seeing the UDR in a new light—not as a nasty, scary foe but as an opportunity for growth and self-determination. Today, rather than finding the UDR's presence in our lives all wrong, we are going to find it *right*.[44]

It is the nature of the UDR to program us to behave a certain way, to get us to believe certain things, to want certain things, and to invest our energy in what it defines as success. The net result of complying with the UDR is, for most of us, a growing sense of discomfort, depletion, anxiety, confusion, and helplessness (as described in part 2, "The Making of a Healthy Deviant").

But at some point on this downward spiral, we either hit bottom and bounce, or we wake up to the fact that we are falling and employ some creative form of self-arrest (like this 14-Day Healthy Deviant Adventure). Or, alternatively, we die. And in all but the last case (where none of us can be certain of what happens), there is an exciting, exhilarating opportunity—the opportunity to radically alter your relationship to the UDR in such a way that it winds up bringing out the best and strongest in you.

How do you do that? First (and rather counterintuitively), you cease seeing the UDR as the enemy. Instead, you begin seeing it as some combination of an inscrutable Zen martial-arts master, a sly trickster, a spiritual drill sergeant, a sucker-punching sparring partner, a dark-side fairy godmother, and a wild and mysterious tango instructor.

The UDR's job is to challenge you, teach you, make you stronger, help you discover your innate gifts, and not let you get away with slacking. It provides you with trials and tribulations. It sends you off on wild goose chases. It tempts you, trips you, flips you, and insists that you get back up again. It presents you with riddles and puzzles and mazes, and never tells you when you are getting it right. It grips you tightly, pulls you off balance, and then pushes you fiercely backward. It gets you drunk, convinces you to tell all your embarrassing secrets, and then ridicules you in public. It leans against the mirrors of the dance studio, smoking a cigarette, and demands that you perform a complex sequence of dance steps again, again, again. It rolls its eyes and snidely laughs at you while you try.

The UDR can make you feel had, beaten, hopeless, defeated, like you are losing your mind. It can make you feel like the whole effort is way too hard, and not worth the bother. It can predispose you to bemoaning your fate and feeling (understandably) sorry for yourself.

Look, it's okay to feel defeated and sorry for yourself sometimes. Just know that it will likely take you further down your downward spiral. Which is fine, because either way, you will eventually bounce, self-arrest, or die.

You know the fastest way to stop spiraling downward? Instead of finding everything unfair and wrong, you can accept it for what it is and find it *right*. Wha?! Find all of this struggle and suffering right? Yes. Perhaps better than right: Perfect. Because even as the UDR subjects you to all this confusion and humiliation, the UDR is making you stronger. In the process of breaking you down, it is also giving you all the information and training you need to outsmart it, to outmaneuver it, and, eventually, as a once-naive apprentice, to take the pebble from its hand.

You stop losing and start winning in relation to the UDR the moment you decide that this is what is going on, that this is just how it is, and thus precisely how it should be. The brilliant Byron Katie calls this creative, constructive, acceptance-based approach to living "loving what is." But even if you don't love how things are right now, you can use this present reality to your advantage to become a bigger, better, more distilled, and extraordinary version of yourself.

Essentially, as long as you are staying ahead of the damage (which you do via Preemptive Repair), what doesn't kill you can make you smarter, stronger, and more damn-the-torpedoes determined. Even as the UDR irritates and oppresses you, it can also inspire and provoke you—to experiment, to rise to the challenge, to take some risks, and to let your Healthy Deviant freak flag fly.

Remember that every day is an opportunity to change the rules of the game. You change those rules, indelibly, as you perform your Renegade Rituals. With each daring repetition, you become wiser, clearer, more skilled, more deft, more unbreakable. In the words of Nassim Taleb, you become "anti-fragile." So today, in the service of your own anti-fragility, what can you find right with yourself and the world?

Nicely done. Well played. Keep going.

Cultivate Willingness

But by my love and hope I beseech you:
Do not throw away the hero in your soul!
Hold holy your highest hope!
—FRIEDRICH NIETZSCHE, *THUS SPOKE ZARATHUSTRA*

One popular characterization of insanity describes it as doing the same thing over and over again, but expecting to get a different result. Well, that particular brand of insanity is hardwired into the Unhealthy Default Reality's (UDR's) automatic programming.

The UDR is designed to get us to do the same (unhealthy) things over and over again, without much thinking about it. And, as noted in part 1, the UDR is also wired up to endlessly sabotage our conscious efforts to change.

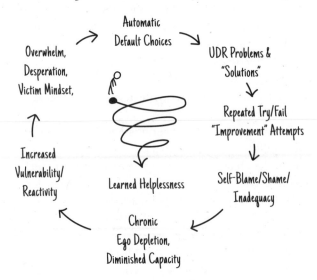

Vicious Cycle of the Unhealthy Default Reality

Automatic Default Choices

UDR Problems & "Solutions"

Repeated Try/Fail "Improvement" Attempts

Self-Blame/Shame/ Inadequacy

Chronic Ego Depletion, Diminished Capacity

Learned Helplessness

Increased Vulnerability/ Reactivity

Overwhelm, Desperation, Victim Mindset,

We saw how this works in part 1:

- The UDR's continuous depletion of our attention, energy, clarity, and self-regard all powerfully undermine the resource we think of as "willpower."

- That wholesale depletion leads, in turn, to numerous failed attempts at change, which in turn give rise to a state of "learned helplessness."

- That state makes us disinclined to invest in any substantive new change efforts, and less capable of following through with the ones we latch onto.

Dah! So how can we break this vicious cycle?

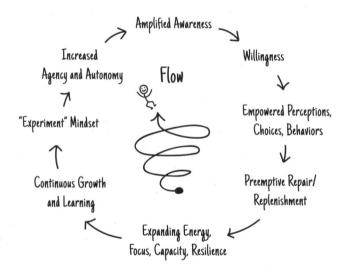

Virtuous Cycle of Healthy Deviance

One helpful approach involves swapping willpower for willingness.

Here's the problem with what we think of as our "will." It's inclined toward being an asshole. It often acts like an arrogant, blustery, hard-driving taskmaster obsessed with a narrowly defined idea of success. The will tends to think it has all the answers, and it doesn't relish asking for feedback or directions.

Willingness, on the other hand, is full of open-minded inquiries, like: How might I go about getting started? How are things going? What would happen if I tried this? What would be most helpful now?

The will says, "Onward at all costs!" Willingness says, "Let's take this a day at a time."

Unlike the will, willingness doesn't get a lot of airtime in our culture. It comes across as too passive, perhaps, too cooperative, too eager to please, too ... feminine. But when it comes to shifting personal behavior and establishing new habits, willingness tends to be a much better and more reliable partner. Call your willingness to you whenever you need it, and it will appear.

In breaking away from the UDR, it's essential we cultivate not just the willingness to do (or not do) certain things, but also the willingness to notice and then more deeply investigate how we do or don't succeed in those endeavors.

The great thing about seeing your chosen change efforts through the lens of willingness is that even if you fail at something on any given day, you can still succeed in learning something valuable that empowers you to succeed the next day.

For example, one thing I used to do a lot (during the "Darkness" period of my Healthy Deviant Hero's Journey) was to eat in the car. I had a long commute, and after a stressful day, eating snacks on the way home felt like a comforting thing to do. I would mindlessly put food in my mouth while I drove, often devouring far more than made any sense relative to my actual level of hunger. Then I'd feel awful about myself. It was a habit I'd tried hard to break by force of will, but I found this particular change didn't respond well to willpower because by the end of the day, I was so depleted and hangry that I didn't have any.

Here's how I used willingness to change it instead. First I asked, "Am I willing to change this?" The answer was yes—with a side of panic and doubt. The truth was, I wasn't yet ready to give it up, and I was afraid that if I tried, I'd fail.

So then I asked, "Am I willing to explore and experiment a bit in the service of changing this habit, or at least understanding it better?" Here, the answer was a solid yes—with a side of excitement. I actually felt energized to explore it! (Biofeedback tip: When you feel an energetic shift like this—whether a rise or fall of energy, a hopeful fluttering or a sinking in your gut—pay attention!)

Then came a series of exploratory questions:

What are the feelings that lead me to want to eat in the car?

- Feeling physically and mentally worn out, overstimulated, and emotionally on edge.

- Wanting to shut down, but feeling like I have to keep going because I still have so much to do.

- Finally feeling free of the pressures and constraints of work, and wanting to get away with doing whatever I want to do.

- Being hungry and suffering from low-blood sugar from having endured a zillion back-to-back meetings not having eaten since lunch.

- Feeling robbed of meaning and satisfaction in my daily experience and thus feeling sad, drained, and resentful.

What are the patterns and experiences that lead up to me being in that depleted, vulnerable, or reactive state?

- Working long hours without a break.
- Not eating healthy snacks before I get really hungry.
- Not prioritizing or feeling that I have really earned pleasure.

What could I do differently so that I might produce a different, better end-of-day experience?

- Take more breaks.
- Take on less work.
- Eat some healthy snacks in the midafternoon.
- Seek out and enjoy more pleasurable, self-sustaining experiences.
- Get some hot herbal tea to drink on my way home.
- Put a reminder in my car to treat myself kindly and with respect.
- If I'm hungry, consider stopping at the co-op for a healthy snack and eating it while sitting down at a table.

Then I asked:

Am I willing to experiment with doing some of those things (or other things I come up with as alternatives)?

- Yes, as long as they don't wear me out further.

Am I willing to pay attention to the results of my experiments?

- Yes, now that I am thinking of them as experiments, I'm curious to see what happens.

All of that was good. There was one more question nagging at me, though: "Am I willing to look at the underlying belief that has had me operating in the self-destructive ways I have been?"

Hmmm. That took some more self-questioning, not all of which was comfortable. But eventually, I did the deep dive and came up with what felt like a true and compelling answer. Underneath this particular compulsive behavior was a stubborn, semi-conscious belief I had long held about needing to do more, to be more, to achieve more in order to be worthy and good. It was a belief about my value coming from what I accomplish, and how perfect, impressive, admirable, and worthy I appeared to others, rather than who I actually was.

When I looked at that, I realized that this was a belief worth examining more closely, because I could see it was probably at the core of not just this one self-destructive pattern, but most of my other self-sabotaging tendencies, too.

If you are interested in doing the deeper work of that last step, I strongly recommend using the "immunity to change" method and the handy "immunity map" described by Robert Kegan, PhD, and Lisa Lahey, PhD, in their terrific book *Immunity to Change.*

In my experience, willpower won't help you go this deep. It doesn't have the patience. And that's just one reason that, over time, I've found willingness to be a far better and more reliable ally. Leaning too heavily on my will, even when it works, brings out the negative and self-critical in me. And research suggests that this is true for many of us (for more on that, google the *Scientific American* article "The Willpower Paradox").

Willpower talks a tough game, but it hates losing—so much so that it is prone to taking its ball and going home just as things are getting interesting. Willingness, meanwhile, sees every "lost" round as an opportunity to sharpen skills, strategy, and awareness (remember how the UDR often shows up as an inscrutable Zen martial-arts master?).

Willingness, in short, is all about learning and growing. Willingness is intrinsically motivating, meaning it elicits the desire to act from within you. And that's why it is at the center of Healthy Deviance, the definition of which begins with "the willingness to defy cultural norms and assumptions."

Today, are you willing to experiment with doing some things differently? Or even just willing to become willing? Are you willing to pay attention to what happens when you do or don't do these things? Are you willing to look at *how* you go about doing or not doing them?

Start by applying willingness to your Renegade Rituals. Which of them are you willing to do today? Call your willingness to you whenever you need it, and it will appear.

DAY 5

Call BS

Being mad is correct; being mad is American;
being mad can be joyful and productive and connective.
Don't ever let them talk you out of being mad again.

—REBECCA TRAISTER

Really?! That is the response I have whenever I flip through most health and fitness magazines, watch television, stumble across fitspo social media posts, read the ingredients on popular food products, or do business with the conventional health-care system. These things tend to offend my Healthy Deviant sensibilities.

My body is supposed to look like that?! This crap is supposed to pass for food? I have to spend all this money and time interacting with a soul-killing bureaucracy only to have some supposed expert tell me they don't know what is wrong with me, that there's no known cause and no known cure, but here's a prescription for a drug that will suppress the symptoms and make matters worse?!

Really?! *Aaaggghh!* What a load of BS!

This stuff makes me mad. Sometimes it makes steam come out my ears. Sometimes it makes me shake my fist. Sometimes it makes me want to simultaneously laugh and cry in exasperation. Almost always, it makes me want to call BS on some aspect of our culture that is messing with my body-mind and my life chances.

Calling BS is really just calling out what is not working. It's saying, "No. Nope. Nice try, Unhealthy Default Reality, but I'm not having it."

The BS in question could be a message, an idea, an implication, an object, a belief, or a whole prescribed way of life. It can be anything that sets you up to fail; anything that tries to separate you from your self-respect, your money, your love, your attention, your choices, or your time; anything that robs you of your Healthy Deviant vitality and autonomy.

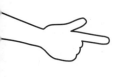

The Unhealthy Default Reality is pretty much made up of wall-to-wall, floor-to-ceiling BS.

But since the BS-production machine of the Unhealthy Default Reality (UDR) is forever operating in the background, cranking out BS night and day, it can be hard to see. Make no mistake, though, the BS is there, making a small number of people a whole lot of money and netting some large, faceless organizations a whole lot of power. All that BS has an important job: Siphoning off your energy, attention, resources, and resilience, and funneling them into the UDR machine, rendering you ever more vulnerable, and making the UDR ever-harder to oppose or resist.

You know what helps you see the UDR and its bottomless BS more clearly? Anger. Yes, I know, anger gets a bad rap in our culture. And we all know why: When it becomes unconscious and out of balance, anger kills and destroys. Still, I think it has a proper place in our lives. Particularly when we are waking up to our present circumstances within the UDR and trying to find our way out of it.

Anger borne of frustration or exasperation with injustice, unfairness, ugliness, greed, cruelty, needless destruction, suffering, waste, and other forms of BS can be a righteous, worthwhile thing. Anger—the kind that calls BS on misery—can be clarifying, energizing, and galvanizing. Like fear, anger can momentarily focus our attention in useful ways. As a short-term tool, as a passageway to greater clarity, it has utility. Of course, when relied on too heavily and too frequently, it can also become a toxic liability. So, it's helpful to understand the proper use and direction of anger.

One of my wise teachers, Cat Thompson (EmotionalTechnologies.com), once told me, "Anger tells you when a boundary has been stepped on, or stepped over." Cat taught me that clear, balanced, healthy anger energy is sacred-warrior energy. That kind of warrior energy is not about fighting and attacking and wounding; it is about choosing, protecting, and safeguarding what matters most to us. The image I have when I think of balanced anger energy is of a calm, strong, centered goddess dressed all in white and holding a tall, richly decorated bronze spear. She is standing outside of a sacred temple, guarding the door. It's her job to protect that temple. And it is her job to call BS on whatever does not belong within it.

This anger-warrior goddess sees all and knows all. You do not get past her without clear intentions. You don't go past her goofing off, or speaking nonsense, or stumbling drunk, or screaming profanities, or wearing headphones, or playing games on your handheld.

She doesn't try to beat you up or poke at you or humiliate you for no good reason. She simply reminds you that you are entering a sacred space, and she doesn't let you pass until you are ready to conduct yourself with clear purpose and proper respect. If necessary, she will rap her spear on the ground to get your attention. If that doesn't work, she will use her spear to block your path. If you try and sneak or lie to get past her, she will matter-of-factly call BS on whatever nonsense you are spewing her way.

I think that right now we need this kind of balanced anger energy—at least in small doses. We need it to help us protect the temples of our body-minds, and our lives. Within the context of the unscrupulous and unbounded UDR, a healthy dose of balanced anger is a good thing to have at your disposal. So today, we are going to keep a lookout for the BS the UDR is constantly cranking out, and we're going to call it when we see it.

Watch for it in the media, in retail locations, in corporate speak. Watch for it in the artifice of advertising. Watch for it in the ideas you carry about yourself and your life that make you feel inherently flawed and not good enough. Watch for it in the assumptions about what you have to be and do and accomplish just to be okay. Watch for it in your own excuses for treating yourself less than kindly.

If you feel a surge of righteous anger when confronted with BS, consider it an indicator, an emergency flare of sorts. Look for the boundary that is being stepped on or stepped over. Wave your fist in exasperation if you need to.

Next, see if you can find both the BS and your pissed-off reaction to it *right* (review day 3 for more on that). What opportunity does the BS give you to solidify a weak boundary, to reclaim your waking state, to grow your mojo, or to learn a new skill?

The BS is relentless and ubiquitous. The more you look for it, the more you will see, and the more you see it for what it is, the less power it will have over you. This is the sort of paradox you must learn to live with in order to outwit the UDR. It is what it is. A lot of it is ugly. A lot of it makes it way harder than it has to be to get and stay healthy. It's okay if all of that makes you mad.

Now, what can you do with all that righteous, balanced, warrior-goddess anger? Set better boundaries. Fine-tune your BS detector. Muster your dignity. Engage in Amplified Awareness, Preemptive Repair, and Continuous Growth and Learning. Affirm your right to just be. Command respect by treating yourself with respect. Redirect your sense of frustration and outrage toward doing what you can do to get stronger and clearer. Starting with your Renegade Rituals.

Remember, you take the wind out of our culture's BS in every moment you see it, see through it, name it, and call it what it is. Every time you point it out so others can see it too. Keep seeing it. Keep pointing it out. Look around and see if you can spot some now.

DAY 6

Ask for What You Want

The true focus of revolutionary change is never
merely the oppressive situations that we seek to escape,
but that piece of the oppressor which is planted deep within us.

—AUDRE LORDE

The Unhealthy Default Reality (UDR) presents you with an endless array of unhealthy and largely automatic, default choices. It proposes a running menu of bad-to-worse options with strong incentives for you to choose among them, quickly, without giving it too much thought. The UDR is the behavior-manipulating equivalent of Instagram advertising linked to Amazon Prime with drone delivery—you see it, you click it, and it's yours. Even if it later gives you a nasty case of buyer's remorse.

Healthy Deviance requires looking beyond the evident and easily accessible options. It requires listening beyond the screaming voices that say, "Pick me! Pick me!" (or, just as often, "Tolerate me! Settle for me!") to instead request what serves you, what empowers you, what the most wise and awake version of you prefers.

In everyday terms, this might mean refusing to be limited by the options on an actual restaurant menu and instead special ordering something that can be cobbled together from the best available whole-food ingredients. But it can also mean looking beyond the default "menu" of choices our society presents us with, from prescribed career paths to preordained relationship paths, from conventional definitions of success to idealized, look-alike notions of beauty.

It can mean noticing what is not currently working for or appealing to you, and seeking to have it changed. It can be noticing what is currently strengthening or delighting you, and deciding to go for more of that. Asking for what you want might mean requesting that a blaring television be turned down or off. It might mean subbing a side of dark greens for toast. It might mean negotiating for a raise or a more flexible work schedule. It might mean asking for more time to yourself or advocating for a deeper and more intimate relationship with your partner.

Asking for what you want and need to be healthy and happy is a Healthy Deviant thing to do. Asking doesn't necessarily mean you'll get it, of course, but the simple act of formulating and making a request can work miracles in the quest to redefine your relationship with the UDR. Here are some things Healthy Deviants tend to ask for:

- Adjustments to their work and home environments that make healthy choices easier and more convenient.

- Access to better, safer, more ecologically sound products.

- Support from friends, partners, and family members in helping them stick to health-supporting patterns and plans.

- Time and space to take care of themselves and pursue goals that matter.

- Minimized exposure to situations and stimuli that drain, distract, derail, or disturb them.

- Opportunities to try or access experiences they think they might enjoy.

- The right to opt-out of experiences that inflame, irritate, deplete, or endanger them.

- Respect for the healthy priorities, boundaries, and structures that sustain them (e.g., no electronics in the bedroom).

- Options and alternatives they don't see offered but hope might be made available.

- Second and third medical opinions; access to integrative, functional practitioners and root-cause approaches to health concerns.

- More information, more perspective, more context, more data.

- Honest feedback, patience, open-mindedness, and support from others.

- The chance to try something different and to see how it goes.

- Forgiveness for unintended screw-ups, negative outcomes, and experiments gone wrong.

- Acceptance and understanding when they change their mind or decide to change course.

- Escapes and recovery breaks from situations that aren't working for them or that they don't feel equipped to handle.

- Increased access and opportunities to experience the things that bring them meaning, pleasure, joy, strength, and satisfaction.

- To be seen and appreciated for who they are—and to see others that same way.

DAY 6

There's more, of course, and every Healthy Deviant is different. But the common "asks" from Healthy Deviants are for things that help them rise to the challenge of being a healthy person in an unhealthy world. They are proposals for creative solutions that support Amplified Awareness, Preemptive Repair, and Continuous Growth and Learning. They are departures from the status quo that stretch and challenge the status quo.

All that stretching and challenging benefits not just the Healthy Deviants who ask for what they want, but also all the Healthy Deviants who follow in their footsteps. Consider how hard it was to eat gluten-free a couple decades ago or to find skincare products without parabens. It got easier because enough of us asked. Let's keep on asking.

When you feel afraid to ask, go back and read "Day 2: Gather Courage," and "Day 4: Cultivate Willingness." When somebody says no, or you can't get the change you want, go back and read "Day 3: Find Things Right."

Consider three things you could ask for that would make your life better, easier, or more beautiful in some way:

- _____

- _____

- _____

One great thing to ask for is the space, time, and support you need to do your Renegade Rituals. You know the best person to ask for that space, time, and support? You.

DAY 7

Celebrate Small Successes

You're entirely bonkers. But I'll tell you a secret.
All the best people are.

—LEWIS CARROLL, *ALICE'S ADVENTURES IN WONDERLAND*

Okay, let's assume you've been doing this Healthy Deviant Adventure thing for a week. By now you have probably run into your share of problems. You've likely run smack into the Unhealthy Default Reality's (UDR's) blockades and elephant traps, and come up against your own resistance. Maybe you've encountered other people's judgments, discouragements, or ridicule.

More than once, even if you posted Healthy Deviant signage all over the place, you have probably forgotten you were even doing this Healthy Deviant Adventure program. Maybe you're three days behind where you think you're supposed to be. Or maybe before you even had a chance to get off course, you got totally fed up and decided to hurl this book across the room. Maybe you quit the program in disgust, abandoned it in defeat, or gave it a sort of half-hearted try but lost steam somewhere around the middle of day 2 and decided, "Meh. I've got too much going on. I'll do this some other time."

It doesn't matter. If you are reading this now—or even if you aren't actually *reading* the book now, but your eyes just happened to glimpse this page as you were picking the book up off the floor from where you hurled it days ago, or from where it fell when you knocked it off the table while dusting or reaching for a bottle of wine—I'm going to encourage you to celebrate. Here's why: You are alive. You are sentient. You have choices. Those are things worth celebrating!

Speaking of choices, remember that Zen saying, "How you do anything is how you do everything"? This would be a good time to look at how you've been doing, or not doing, this Healthy Deviant Adventure. It would be a good time to consider how are you doing, or not doing, your daily readings and your Renegade Rituals?

Because however you have been approaching this book and this program (dutifully, grudgingly, lackadaisically?) is probably also how you tend to approach a bunch of other things, especially the things you believe to be good for you or that you think you "should" do. If you can look at that, consider how that might be true, and perhaps pull some insights from that, you are doing this program perfectly.

I'd also like to invite you to reflect on how you are doing as we near the end of phase 1. Whatever you are thinking about this whole concept of Healthy Deviance, and however you are responding or reacting to this program, how are you doing in your body-mind right now? How are you doing relative to your own baseline normal and relative to when you started reading and thinking about this stuff?

You don't have to say you are doing better if you aren't, or even that you've noticed a change. There's no right answer here. What I'm hoping you might consider is what the experience of doing or not doing this book has been like. I'd also like to invite you to consider what (if anything) you are feeling willing and energized to do now in the service of your health, your energy, your sanity.

If you can feel any willingness at all, if you've been willing to experiment with even one small idea I've offered you, or to entertain an insight or question of your own while you were reading or practicing any of this, I'd consider that a success, and I'd encourage you to celebrate it. If you've made even one slightly healthier choice during the course of this program, I'd encourage you to celebrate doubly.

The UDR has a sneaky way of making you feel like you are forever failing, struggling, falling short. Whenever you're approaching one of its infernal goal lines, the goal moves. So most of us never really get to feel we've succeeded. We tire of trying and failing. And this sets us up for that whole learned help-lessness dynamic I described in part 1. That dynamic, as you now know, is one of the UDR's most insidious traps.

If you're still hanging in here with me, it means you haven't fallen for that trap. If you are still reading, that shows willingness, agency, and initiative. It speaks of your ability to focus your attention. These are Healthy Deviant capacities you can build on. These are things worth celebrating.

As I noted in part 3, when I first described the Nonconformist Competencies (Amplified Awareness, Preemptive Repair, Continuous Growth and Learning), these are not things you master all at once. Nor are they things that you are ever "done" practicing. They aren't things you ever perfect, graduate from, or put behind you. Rather, they are an abiding set of interests and skills you steadily develop over time, with directed attention and intentional practice. So if you've been doing even a little of that, with or without this book's help, you are doing well. You are on your way. You are authoring your Healthy Deviant Hero's Journey as you see fit, as only you can do.

And now, you have a decision to make. You can either proceed to phase 2 of this program, or you can go back to the beginning of phase 1 and approach it with fresh energy and attention. Please note that phase 2 is not better than phase 1. It isn't necessarily harder (although it does offer some additional challenges designed to get you to notice some new things about yourself and your relationship with the UDR). The first thing to notice, even as we approach phase 2, is how you relate to the idea of progress in the context of a multiphase plan—even one as random as a Healthy Deviant Adventure.

Do you feel pressure to advance? Is this another opportunity for perceived success or failure? Are you hungry for variety? Does the idea of repeating phase 1 make you squirm? Are you waiting to get to the "good part" and impatient for dramatic results? Are you eager to get to closure on this thing? Or do you feel like you didn't do phase 1 well enough, and thus need to repeat it until you get it right?

Whatever your tendency to think or feel or be inclined to do one thing or another, just notice that about yourself—and again, celebrate. Maybe reach around and pat yourself on the back, or run yourself a bath, or go sit in the sunshine for a moment and just reflect with pride on the fact that you can notice.

Take a look back, too, and see how you did or did not do various Renegade Rituals. Take a moment to review your Daily Deviance Journal Pages. How many of them did you fill out, and with what level of detail? Putting your attention on your choices, your actions, and your experiences. Observing your patterns with curiosity. Investigating your inner and outer workings. These are the skills of a Healthy Deviant. And you are practicing them now.

This week's themes (waking up, gathering courage, cultivating willingness, finding things right, calling BS, asking for what you want, and celebrating small successes) are the themes of a Healthy Deviant lifetime. So it doesn't really matter whether you ever move onto phase 2. This is the official end of phase 1, though. This is a great time to pause and reflect. What small successes can you recognize from the past week, whether moments of noticing, conscious choice, insights, or just the willingness to keep going? Name three:

- _____

- _____

- _____

This is also a great time to practice your Renegade Rituals with special attention, noticing whether they have gotten any easier to do, whether your experience with them is any different than when you began this cycle.

Either way, know this: You're doing something almost nobody does. Give yourself some credit for that. (Don't expect the UDR to do it for you.)

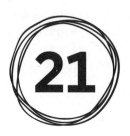

21

PHASE 2

Raise Your Game

People wish to be settled;
only as far as they are unsettled
is there any hope for them.

—RALPH WALDO EMERSON

DAY 8

Abandon Victim Thinking

Character—the willingness to
accept responsibility for one's own life—
is the source from which self-respect springs.

—JOAN DIDION

If dealing with the oppressive assaults of the Unhealthy Default Reality (UDR) sometimes makes you feel downtrodden, that's understandable. The UDR can be a real beast, and because it operates covertly, 24/7, it's only a matter of time until it either catches us off guard or wears down our resistance. And the moment we lower our defenses, the UDR does its best to *keep* them down.

We may start feeling like no matter how hard we work, nothing will ever change. We may start hating our bodies, our circumstances, our lives. We may feel small, sad, and helpless—like we've got the whole world on our shoulders and we've been saddled with more problems than we can ever hope to fix. That suits the Unhealthy Default Reality just fine. Because when we feel victimized and desperate, we accept default choices more easily. We consume more and create less. We look to authorities for answers and solutions rather that innovating and experimenting on our own.

When you're feeling depleted and beaten down, you're typically not inclined to begin questioning, reimagining, or disrupting the systems around you. You're just trying to get by. Victim mindsets tend to be self-perpetuating, and they can be tricky to extract yourself from. So if you're deep into wallowing at the moment, I'm not going to tell you that you have to stop. Just keep in mind that "poor me" is unlikely to get you anywhere you really want to go.

That said, I reserve my right to have a good whine-and-moan session now and then—about how hard everything is, how nothing ever works out, how "I don't know how" or "don't think I can," and how this or that thing always happens to me. Wah, wah, wah. I sometimes find that slogging around in my own self-pity serves as a much needed release. Plus, if I stay at my own pity party for long enough, I tend to get bored with it. At some point, I recognize that for things to evolve, I have to quit my complaining and start advocating for the changes I want to see, both in my circumstances and in myself.

When faced with a big, scary, or oppressive problem, I am a big believer in following T. Harv Eker's advice to decide that you can be "bigger than the problem." One way to get bigger than your problems, even if you don't yet know how to solve them, is simply to assume a higher-level, more objective view of them. I sometimes like to visualize myself as a sort of modern-day, female Sherlock Holmes—an objective sleuth keenly interested in sorting out precisely how and when poor-little-victimized-me got herself into the sad state of affairs she is currently bemoaning.

When I take close, curious, and courageous inventory of the choices that got me to my victimized state, I often discover that somewhere along the way, I made some choices *to avoid or delay making choices.* Maybe I let other people and institutions evaluate my worth or make my choices for me. Once I start investigating a given situation or problem this way, I often discover that my current victimized state has everything to do with my abdication of my responsibility to myself. Somewhere along the way, I fell under the Unhealthy Default Reality's sway. I got sucked into its programming and prescriptions, or let myself become tangled up in its crazy notions of what is good and right and true.

Deferring to the Unhealthy Default Reality is always dangerous. When we allow it to dictate our plans, restrict our options, and sell us on its definitions of how things should be (or how *we* should be), we generally wind up face down in the dirt, begging for help that never comes. Operating from this place of victimization further depletes us and ratchets our suffering to a new level.

All the while, the Unhealthy Default Reality continues feeding on our misery. But keep in mind, the Unhealthy Default Reality is also giving us an opportunity to get stronger, to get bigger, to rise to a new level of mastery and capacity in which we can "take the pebble from its hand."[45]

So today, let us pick ourselves up, dust ourselves off, and embrace our training. Let us throw off the chains of our victimhood and examine them for clues. Where did they come from? How long have we been wearing them? What excuses have they given us for staying where we are, playing it safe, not owning the truth of our own bodies, hearts, and minds? What are we afraid might happen if we left the chains behind?

Today, consider one or more situations in which you have tended to fall into "poor me" thinking or been inclined to inhabit a powerless, victimized state of mind. Locate areas in your life where you are currently thinking, "I can't!" or "I have no choice!" or "I need somebody to save me!" Consider: What more empowered, dignified, and true thing could you be thinking instead? You might try completing some phrases like, "I choose … " or "I am moving toward …" or "I'm excited to learn how to …"

Then perform your Renegade Rituals, and notice that the simple act of redirecting your attention, energy, and moment-by-moment choices is an act of empowered rebellion. In those moments, you are not a victim anymore.

Find Your Edge

Be willing to be uncomfortable.
Be comfortable being uncomfortable.
It may get tough, but it's a
small price to pay for living a dream.

—PETER MCWILLIAMS

The tricky thing about growth is that it always involves some discomfort, even if that discomfort comes entirely from unfamiliarity. In the moment we move from the known to the unknown, from easily within reach to just out of reach, we enter the territory of our growing edge—and man, does that tend to feel like someplace we'd rather not hang out.

This is also true of Healthy Deviance. In the moments we oppose the Unhealthy Default Reality (UDR), question the status quo, or defy any convention we've historically complied with, there are some funky moments of discomfort. When those moments happen to me, I consider them close encounters with my growing edge.

If you want to find your growing edge really quickly, try standing on one foot for a moment. The moment you start to wobble, you've found your growing edge. This is the place of your current capacity to balance on one foot. It is a function of your current neurological wiring, focus, proprioception, biomechanics, and muscle development. No wobble? Lean far enough in any direction that you *do* wobble. Find that place where you start to lose your balance, and you'll have found the meeting ground between what you can currently do and what you can't—yet.

The point is, we all have a wobble point. We can stay safely within its territory, in which case we will not discover new ground, or we can reach beyond our current zone of comfort and competency and go someplace we haven't. When you find your current edge, you'll also probably connect with the distinct feeling of being out of control, of being momentarily at odds with yourself, of not knowing how, of being at risk of failing at something, and thus wanting to quit.

Keep at the balancing exercise for a while, for example, and as your muscles, focus, and patience all tire of the challenge, you'll think, "Okay, I get it. This is hard and annoying, and I really don't want to do this anymore."

In the moment just before you give up, though—in that split second between seeing if you can and finding that you can't or won't—there is a strange, extraordinary magic. And if you can hold onto that moment just a wee tiny bit longer than you feel inclined to, you'll discover something notable:

What you believed to be your edge is not. At least, it's not anymore.

Because as you inhabit the space in between can and can't, will and won't, that space expands, if even by a tiny, microcosmic amount. Remain at your edge just long enough to notice it, and in that moment of noticing and naming, you'll be getting stronger, you'll be building capacity and equanimity. Go to the frontier of your current edge, and you'll learn that frontier is further out there than you think. And the more you explore in that edge region of yours, the more skilled you will become at navigating it with confidence, even pleasure.

Flirting with your current edge is basically free, live entertainment. Here are a few fun places to explore it:

Food: Put something edible in front of you that you would like to eat. Decide that you are, in fact, going to eat it, but there's no rush to do so. You can look at it, smell it. You can just notice and be with the feeling of being about to eat something. Perhaps this is not an experience you would normally extend, but since you can eat it any time you want, there's no harm in giving it another second or two. Or three or four. Notice the feelings and thoughts that come up as you wrestle with the decision of whether to bite into it now … or now … or now.

Movement: Jog, jump, skip, or walk quickly until you feel inclined to stop—either because you are out of breath or because your muscles are tiring. Then decide to take another step or two. Are you at your edge now? Is it really all that different than the earlier moment you wanted to stop? Could you do one more? How about three more or five more or ten? Notice the feelings and thoughts that come up as you wrestle with the decision of whether to stop now … or now … or now.

Meditation: Sit quietly with your eyes closed or gazing at a single spot and keep your attention only on your breath. Notice your first inclination to stop. Then sit for just a moment longer, maybe the length of a breath or two. Or three or four. Totally up to you. Now, knowing it's just for the span of one more breath, or whenever you decide, could you sit for just that tiny spell longer? Notice the feelings and thoughts that come up as you wrestle with the decision of whether to break away from your meditation now ... or now ... or now.

Shower: Experiment with having the water just a tiny bit warmer or cooler than you like it. Go back and forth between the two extremes, finding temperatures that are not excruciating, but just enough too-warm or too-cold to be a tiny bit uncomfortable. Take note of your preferences, of the exquisite sensitivity of your skin, and what a tiny margin there is, on both the hot and cold ends, between the temperatures you prefer and the temperatures you do not. Could you tolerate it just a little bit warmer or cooler, or sit with the not-so-comfortable temperature just a second or two longer? Notice the feelings and thoughts that come up as you wrestle with the decision of whether to put the temperature back to precisely where you like it now ... or now ... or now.

In each case, avoid pushing or enduring to the point you take on huge tension and stress or freak yourself out. Just hang out in that in-between place for as long as you are learning something new about yourself and your own reactions.

You'll notice something interesting is happening in all these experiments, and once you do, you'll find it's a phenomenon you can begin playing with and practicing in a thousand different ways. You can wash your hands for a moment longer than you normally would, breathe just a little more deeply than you typically do, wait one second longer to respond to an impulse, to react to a craving, to decide yes or no.

Pushing beyond the habitual, the comfortable, and the currently easy is a great developmental practice for all forms of Healthy Deviance. Because breaking from social norms and automatic, unhealthy default choices involves doing just that, over and over and over again.

So, how can you find, experience, and extend your growing edge today? Try it with one of the experiments above, with your Renegade Rituals, or in any situation where you're intent on creating positive change.

DAY 10

Renegotiate Reality

Sandra: Well, Murray, to sort of return to reality for a moment ...
Murray: I'll go, but only as a tourist.
—FROM THE 1965 FILM, *A THOUSAND CLOWNS*

Our lives reflect our agreements—both conscious and unconscious. Look around at your current reality, and you'll see evidence of what you have either tacitly or explicitly agreed to do. That includes what you've agreed to believe and value, how you've agreed to direct your attention, whom you've agreed to spend time with, and the things in which you've agreed to invest your time, energy, and money.

For better or worse, our society reflects the agreements we are all making collectively. But none of those agreements is etched in stone. I'm a firm believer that when we observe that a particular agreement is not playing out the way we'd hoped, it's perfectly acceptable to go about renegotiating it. Renegotiate enough agreements, and in the process, you'll wind up renegotiating your reality.

For example, at one time, I agreed to spend a lot of time, energy, and money on my appearance because I believed that having the "right" appearance would make me happy. At some point, I unconsciously agreed (as many of us do) that the appearance I would attempt to cultivate would look at lot like the appearance of the women I saw on television and on the covers of magazines. It took me a long time to realize that that effort was thankless and that it was making me miserable. But once I did, I decided to alter my previous agreement. I decided that I would stop watching television, that I would stop having those magazines around my home, and that I would stop giving them my attention when I ran across them in public places.

Then I made a variety of new agreements with myself. Rather than investing my time and money in chasing a particular look, I started defining a more comfortable and expressive style of my own. I started putting less attention on perfecting my appearance and more attention on developing my inner resources, pursuing gratifying relationships, investigating my areas of curiosity, and appreciating the beauty I see all around me. I have found these agreements to be much more rewarding.

The agreements of Healthy Deviants often run counter to the agreements of other people. They may not agree to value the same things, to get with the same programs, or to settle for the same solutions that others do. They often decide to spend their time, attention, money, and effort in radically different ways than the Unhealthy Default Reality (UDR) entices or pressures them to. And they may take all kinds of heat for that.

The Way of the Healthy Deviant involves developing skills that others don't have, defending priorities that others don't care about, and rewriting commitments that most others see as ironclad. The sooner you get good at that, the further you separate your life from the contracts the UDR insists we all sign, the healthier and happier your life will be.

So, how do you renegotiate the agreements you've made in your own life? It starts by valuing your own health, happiness, and autonomy enough to believe they are worth defending. From there, it generally involves a series of "courageous conversations" in which you openly share the ways in which your values and priorities are informing your decisions to call for change.

At work, this may mean renegotiating the requirements of your position, your schedule, or your physical environment in ways that allow you to take better care of yourself. At home, it may mean rethinking the framework of your habits and relationships—from how often you order takeout to whether electronics are allowed in your bedroom. From how you relate during disagreements to where you go on vacation.

You may also wind up renegotiating some things with yourself. That may mean acknowledging that you feel some new desire or priority calling, and that you've decided to heed that call, even if it requires you to move into some uncharted territory and to develop as-yet-undeveloped skills.

There is no shame or failure in renegotiating your agreements. It is, in fact, an act of great integrity, one that puts you into greater alignment with who you are, the life you choose to lead, and the contributions you choose to make while you walk this earthly plane. That doesn't mean it will be easy, of course, or without repercussions. The renegotiation of some agreements, especially those you've never before thought to question, can look like outright rebellion. They can create all sorts of friction and conflict. That's why I suggest starting by renegotiating some smaller commitments first.

The Renegade Rituals are a great way to wade into this sort of renegotiation. They bust you out of ruts in ways that others will inevitably notice and question, giving you an open forum in which to announce the changes you are making in the service of your own well-being. They tend to challenge agreements you may not even realize you have made—to put others' preferences ahead of your own, to do the things that others consider normal, to continue to do things that are breaking you down because, well, that's just what you've always done.

Today, consider one agreement that you've made, knowingly or unknowingly, that you might choose to renegotiate.

DAY 11

Act "As If"

We seldom realize, for example, that our most
private thoughts and emotions are not actually our own.
For we think in terms of languages and images which we
did not invent, but which were given to us by our society.

—ALAN W. WATTS

We humans have a nasty habit of seeing the current version of ourselves as who we really are. We repeatedly practice and perform the role of our current selves with such reliable precision that we don't know how to play any other role or even how to vary our script. In doing what we've always done, of course, we get what we've always gotten. And when we don't like those results, we tend to step into our well-practiced victim role (see "Day 8: Abandon Victim Thinking," above).

The Unhealthy Default Reality (UDR) loves this, because it means we can be relied upon to maintain our passive state of chronic ego depletion and learned helplessness. As our health erodes, and as we accumulate medical diagnoses, we become even more helpless and passive, or we invest ever-greater amounts of time, energy, and money in the ineffective solutions and counterproductive fixes the UDR cranks out. Either way, the UDR wins. If enough of us quit playing along with this routine, the Unhealthy Default Reality would wither and a Healthy Default Reality would take its place. But we're not inclined to do that. Our brains are wired to keep us performing (and thus producing) the status quo.

There's a fascinating branch of neuroscience focused on what's known as brain plasticity. This describes brain's ability to dynamically reshape itself, to lay down new synaptic networks and rearrange old ones based on our current patterns of thought and action. Back in the late 1940s, a neuropsychologist named Donald Hebb observed that within the human brain, "neurons that fire together, wire together." And today, thanks to the miracle of positron emission tomography (PET), we know this is true. The more we think or behave in certain ways, the more we lay down robust neural networks to support those modes of thought and behavior. And the stronger those networks get, the harder it becomes for us to think in new and different ways that might bust us out of our own mental, emotional, and physical ruts.

The 2004 film *What the Bleep Do We Know!?* features a terrific animation that demonstrates exactly how this works. By showing how our synaptic connections physically form and reform to accommodate our brain activity and how our biochemistry responds to our emotional states, it explains how our neuroplasticity can keep us tied to limiting, habitual modes of thought, feeling, and behavior. It also explains how we can leverage our neuroplasticity to set ourselves free from the self-created prisons of our own minds. I strongly recommend watching the whole film, but if you just want to see a few minutes of the animation in question, check out my YouTube channel, where I've saved that segment of video to my Healthy Deviant playlist.

Dr. Joe Dispenza, one of the featured experts who explains this phenomenon in the film, also describes it in much greater detail in his own books, videos, audio lectures, and guided meditations. And once you understand the basic science behind how we can leverage your brain's neuroplasticity to move beyond your current synaptic limitations, you will never view who you really are in quite the same way.

Basically, it comes down to thinking thoughts and performing actions *as if* your chosen realities were already so, and *as if* the changes you desire had already occurred. As you go about practicing that "as if" reality, you begin laying down the new neural networks that support it. Your thoughts create your feelings, and your feelings create biochemical cascades. Those biochemical cascades flip switches in your DNA, shift the behavior of your cells, and ultimately reform your physical cell tissue. In other words, as you shift your brain infrastructure, emotional states, DNA, and cell tissue, you effectively become a different version of yourself. The "as if" version of you increasingly becomes who you really are.

The Three Walks exercise in chapter 18 can give you a good example of how this works. As you inhabit the regal posture and dignified gait of a monarch, you will start to feel more dignified and to think more regal thoughts. As you perform the playful attitude and energy of a happy child, you will likely feel more energetic and entertain more positive thoughts.

So today, consider how you would think and act if you already were a healthy, happy, fully empowered person. How would you stand, sit, and carry yourself? How would you approach the act of eating? How would you care for your body and advocate for your needs? How would you relate to other people? How would you go about your day? Even imagining these scenarios can be powerful, but actually performing them, trying them on in real life, is transformative.

Today, consider where and how you could act as if your Healthy Deviant identity was fully formed. Even if you are doing some less-than-healthy things, imagine how a healthy person would do them. How would a healthy person eat a candy bar, for example? What attitude would they have in choosing and openly enjoying it? List three things you'll do today with a Healthy Deviant attitude (your Renegade Rituals are fair game):

- _____
- _____
- _____

DAY 12

Stake Your Claim

The master's tools will never dismantle the master's house.
—AUDRE LORDE

In a world where chronic illness, fatigue, and depression have become the new normal, it's easy to forget that health is our natural state. It's easy to begin thinking that the goal of vibrant health and energy is beyond reach. Once pronounced ill, many patients quickly become convinced that their disease state is now just part of their life and their identity. They come to believe they cannot expect much more than a treatment plan and some short-term relief from their symptoms. For some, symptom suppression and disease management may be the only alternative. For many, though, it is just the default choice *presented* as the only alternative.

Go to a conventional medical doctor with a typical health complaint and you're likely to be told that it's a common problem among people of your life stage or gender, or a rare and mysterious problem that they don't quite understand. There may be some casting about for the proper, specific diagnoses (to make sure you know it's version B of Malady Problem-itis, not version A). But there likely will be no discussion about how you can reasonably hope to return yourself to a state of optimal health. Because almost nobody is in a state of optimal health these days, neither we nor our doctors often see examples of it in our daily lives. As a result, with time and exposure to the Unhealthy Default Reality (UDR), our expectations for our own health and happiness tend to drift downward.

When I was in my thirties, I developed a case of perioral dermatitis (a common complaint among women of that age). I was offered a prescription cream. Then my eyelashes started falling out. I was given another cream. Neither cream helped much, so I stopped using them. The rash eventually went away, and my eyelashes grew back, but only after I lowered my stress level (by insisting on having more help at work and also taking more breaks throughout the day), lowered my intake of inflammatory foods, and started getting a lot more sleep.

In my late forties, I developed a case of geographic tongue. I was told it was a "benign inflammatory condition" (and evident oxymoron) for which there was no cure, and that I could expect to have it for the rest of my life.

And yet, during a medically supervised, weeklong water fast, it healed completely. Through research and trial-and-error experimentation, I discovered that raw nuts and a few other things I'd been eating frequently had been contributing to the problem.

My partner Alan suffered from excruciating cluster headaches (also known as "suicide headaches") for more than a decade. He was told they were incurable. But then he followed a gluten-free diet and supplementation protocol recommended by functional neurologist David Perlmutter, MD, and inside of three weeks, the headaches were gone. His life was entirely altered by this unexpected remission. Interestingly, when he switched to some cheaper supplements he ordered off the internet, the headaches came back. When he switched to his original brand and source, they disappeared again.

Terry Wahls, MD, a clinical professor of medicine at the University of Iowa, received a diagnosis of multiple sclerosis, widely believed to be an incurable condition that would lead inevitably to declining states of health and mobility. And yet she reversed her supposedly irreversible disease using a nutrient-rich, grain-free, mitochondria-building, mind-body-spirit-healing lifestyle approach that is now being hailed as a huge breakthrough in treating autoimmune conditions of all sorts. (For more on that, read her book, *The Wahls Protocol,* watch her TED Talk, and check out her evolving research at TerryWahls.com.)

I'm not a medical doctor, and I am not going to offer you any personal or professional advice on your current medical conditions. But I will say this. In my immediate circle of friends and family, and in my much wider circle of readers and listeners, I've witnessed all sorts of autoimmune diseases, skin conditions, digestive problems, and even brain problems disappear when the root causes of those conditions were addressed and the entire body-mind system strengthened.

These were not, in the view of the people who experienced them, miracle cures. They were the result of figuring out what was making their body mad, and ceasing to do, host, or endure those things. They were the result of appropriate interventions and adjustments that were, at long last, accomplished—much as the body had long desired.

My point is not that every once in a while, chronic diseases and conditions thought to be incurable turn out not to be. My point, my contention, is that virtually *all* chronic diseases can be reversed, arrested, or at least radically ameliorated, if you can just figure out what has triggered them, remove the triggers, support the body's self-healing capacities, and then give the body's systems the time and resources they need to repair the damage.

Of course, if you believe your health complaints are normal or incurable, you're not going to bother doing all that. Instead, you're going to settle for a vastly lower quality of life. You're going to keep doing the things that are messing with your health, and you're going to start accumulating both diagnoses and disease-management programs. You're going to design your career choices, your financial resources, and your relationships around those limitations.

If you want to have the healthiest body-mind available to you, you have to believe that your body-mind is yours to make or break. You have to defend it against the pronouncements of people (including, potentially, experts and authoritative sources) who are inclined to see you as a diagnosis, and who would have you believe there's little or nothing you can do to improve your own health. You may have to decide you will not be limited by what is covered or reimbursable as part of your health insurance plan.[46] Instead, as I discussed in chapter 4, you have to see your chronic illness or condition as one of many expressions of Pissed-Off Body Syndrome, and figure out what you are doing or not doing (or just plain experiencing as a result of being in this mixed up world of ours) that is pissing it off.

There are many ways of going about this (elimination diets and autoimmune protocols being among the most popular and accessible). The first step is simply staking a claim to your own well-being and deciding you will defend it with everything you've got.

Know that this is a supremely radical, openly defiant, Healthy Deviant thing to do. And if you do it, you must be prepared for people telling you that you are giving yourself and others false hope, or worse. You will hear sick people arguing for their chronically ill identities. You will hear their friends and families insisting that by even suggesting there might be some means of lifestyle-based intervention or reversal, you are victim blaming, and that this is a cruel and shameful thing to do. You will hear droves of conventional doctors insisting that you've been misled by fakers and quacks, that you are practicing medicine without a license, and that you pose a danger to yourself and others.

At this point, you will have a choice: Submit to the ministrations of the Unhealthy Default Reality or buck the system and seek out the Healthy Deviant approaches that work for you. Today, if you're feeling like doing the latter, list one health condition or challenge (from low energy to a persistent rash, ache, pain, mystery ailment, or diagnosed disease state) for which you'd be willing to explore an empowered solution.

Condition you are willing to explore:

_____

Then read a few of the articles listed later in this chapter (in the section called "When You're Freaking Out"). Or fire up a search engine and type in a name or description of that condition along with the terms *functional medicine, lifestyle, epigenetic,* and *root cause* in quotes. See what comes up.

I'm not saying that you can google your way to wellness or even that you need to be fixed. I'm not saying that your pain or illness is your fault. I'm not saying there is a miracle cure in your future. I'm not selling you an instant fix. What I am saying is that you have right and reason to do everything in your power to get and stay as healthy and happy as you choose to be. No matter how incurable you may believe your condition to be, there's probably still a great deal you can do to help your body deal with whatever challenges life has thrown your way, and in the process, to discover more of what makes your life worth living.

DAY 13

——

Expand Your Horizon

Dullness is a disease.

—FREDDIE MERCURY

What does a healthy, happy person look like? It's hard to say, because we live in a culture that presents us with a pretty limited array of visible examples.

The pictures of healthy people we see most often tend to be slender, affluent white people (or light-skinned people of color) with everything arranged just so. They tend to have carefully (yet casually) styled hair, manicured nails, and exceptionally white, straight teeth. They tend to be people with tons of leisure time, in-home gyms, and unfettered access to unspoiled beaches. They tend to be people with clear kitchen counters who dress in wardrobe-styled yoga outfits and live in art-directed homes. They tend to be people without a care in the world, intent on perfecting their already perfect bodies.

There's a funny meme called "women laughing alone with salad" and another called "women struggling to drink water" that will give you a good sense of how these people look. During my early years at *Experience Life,* I sometimes included images like these in the pages of the magazine because I, too, had been brainwashed by our culture into believing this was what health looked like. And because all the vast coffers of stock photography were (and still are) full of them. But I'm here to tell you now:

This is not what health and happiness really look like.

These expressions of health and happiness are not the biggest prizes available to those who seek and embody them. At least, not for most people.

There are all kinds of healthy people out there. People of all colors and stripes, people of all genders and orientations, people of all fashion preferences and predilections, people of all economic strata and diverse political views. There are Healthy Deviants who appear surprisingly conformist, and Healthy Deviants who openly let their freak flag fly.

So it's worth thinking about what your own health and happiness look like to you. And what they feel like. Beyond the appearance of your body, beyond the art direction of your immediate surroundings, what kind of person will you become when you are a healthier, happier version of yourself? What kind of life will you lead? What impact could you have?

Can't see it now? You will.

This is how it works: When we first start imagining what a healthy, happy life might look like and feel like, we can only see so far. But when we get to the horizon we've envisioned, we can perceive a totally different horizon.

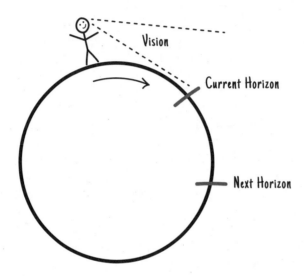

Right now, it may be all about your body. The size and shape you want to be. The amount of weight you want to be able to lift. The number of miles you want to be able to run. But at some point, as your health and happiness improve, you're going to get to a new horizon. And then, you're going to start envisioning and caring about different things.

At some point, the health of your body-mind will become the means to a greater end, some higher purpose or desire or sense of possibility that you may not yet be able to discern. Which is A-okay. Remember, seeing it clearly is the work of some future horizon. But it can also be fun to imagine right now …

- What might I do with myself when I have more energy, focus, clarity?

- How might I show up in the world?

- How will my options expand?

- What larger challenges might I take on?

- What barriers to health might I help to point out or break down?

- What social, environmental, or larger systemic issues could I address?

- Whom else within my circle or community might I be able to help?

Even if right now, you are so sick, tired, and overwhelmed that you can't imagine lifting a finger to take on one more challenge or help anybody but yourself, it can be encouraging to know that you will not always feel that way. Eventually, you will start feeling the truth of that old saying:

If you are not part of the solution, you are part of the problem.

Maybe not this week. Maybe not this month. But at some point, when you are healthy and happy enough to have a surplus of energy and enthusiasm, it will almost certainly happen: You'll want to invest some part of that surplus in addressing the root causes of the problems you have been facing, and that you see others facing, too.

Right now, by addressing your personal health issues, and upgrading the well-being of your body-mind, you are becoming "bigger than the problem." And in the process, you are becoming part of the solution. You are answering the call of the Healthy Deviant Hero's Journey, acquiring heroic gifts—skills and perspectives and capacities—that you will eventually share with others.

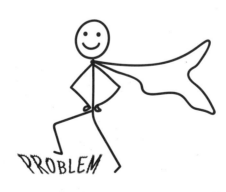

In the moments when you are hating on yourself or mourning the loss of your sugar cereal, these are worthwhile things to remember. These are the horizons that it can be fun to begin scanning for, even if they seem awfully far off right now. Trust they will come into view. It's just a matter of time.

Meanwhile, seizing the opportunities you can to "pay it forward" right now can also bring new energy and satisfaction to your own health-improvement efforts. When you "Ask for What You Want" (Day 6)—whether healthier menu options or better health-care options—you make it easier for others to do the same.

List one thing about the world that drives you crazy. Some form of injustice, waste, or degradation that we could all do without.

_____

Then envision the healthiest possible you perched on top of its vanquished form, hero-cape flying.

That's your new horizon.

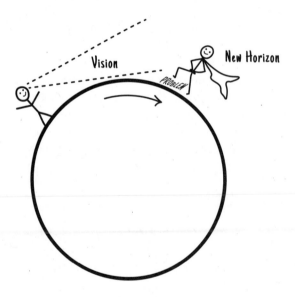

DAY 14

Bask, Beware, Repeat

Success breeds complacency.
Complacency breeds failure.
Only the paranoid survive.

—ANDY GROVE

If you've been going along with this Healthy Deviant Adventure program, and you've been trying on some of the new thoughts and behaviors it recommends, you've probably been making some progress. Maybe you are experiencing some subtle or not-so-subtle shifts in how you feel and how you relate to your world.

You may be thinking, "Hey, this isn't so hard! I think I've got this!"

If so, I'm thrilled, because that is exactly how I had hoped you might feel. And if not, that's entirely okay and understandable, because what I'm inviting you to explore here is not some simple green-juice detox; it's a radical rethinking of your entire life and your relationship to the most dominant and entrenched institutionalized systems around you.

Either way, I want to remind you that the path of the Healthy Deviant is much like the path of everything else in nature: An oscillating wave, a set of cycles that never cease.

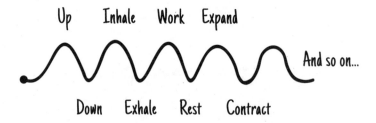

Up   Inhale   Work   Expand

And so on...

Down   Exhale   Rest   Contract

There are ups and downs, moments of victory and defeat, times of expansion and contraction, times of elation and times of "meh." There are times when you feel you have it all figured out and that the Unhealthy Default Reality (UDR) can't touch you. And there are times when the UDR sucker punches you and leaves you sprawled and whimpering on the floor. The experience of a Healthy Deviant embraces all of that, understanding that in the low times, the lift is coming, available, within reach, just around the corner. It comes via Amplified Awareness, Preemptive Repair, Continuous Growth and Learning. It comes via Renegade Rituals and Healthy Deviant Survival Skills.

Along the way, it is good to bask in even the smallest of successes. The conscious commute in which you allowed three cars in front of you *and* smiled at the guy who flipped you off. The first night you decided to keep the television off and realized how pleasant your home can be without it on. The meal in which you never lost consciousness, never stopped breathing, and thus recognized the instant you no longer desired to keep eating. The moment you were brushing your teeth by candlelight and thought, *I could do with more candlelight in my life.*

It's also good to be aware that you will have some less glorious moments. Moments when you move beyond your edge, eat the donut, and decide to loathe yourself for hours afterward. Moments when you find yourself envying somebody else's body and entirely ignoring the dignity and majesty of your own. Moments when you are so loaded down with the shoulds and have-tos of the Unhealthy Default Reality that your victimized self begins calling the shots.

In those less glorious moments, here's what I want you to keep in mind:

In states of chronic depletion and overwhelm, you are a terrible judge of your own capacity and your inherent worth.

Perhaps you overestimated what you could manage in this moment. Perhaps you let your guard down. Perhaps you just ascended to a new level of play and are still learning the rules of the game. It's all okay. This does not mean you are incapable of rising to the challenge. It means you are in the process of rising to the challenge. And now you've got some new information to integrate into your plan.

Perform a Renegade Ritual. Evaluate whether there's a Nonconformist Competency you could draw on, or use this as an opportunity to strengthen it. Find some way to temporarily retreat from the UDR to rebuild your resources, even if that means sneaking into a bathroom stall and doing some deep breathing. Then reemerge, intent on bringing your Healthy Deviant self to the party. Begin the climb to your next top-performance peak with the goal of experiencing it in all its glory.

Bask, beware, repeat.

Prepare to do that again. And again. And again.

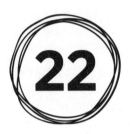

Your Healthy Deviant Toolkit

I've learned that you shouldn't go through life
with a catcher's mitt on both hands;
you need to be able to throw something back.

—MAYA ANGELOU

Is this experience over? Hardly. What I've gathered for you here (and also online at HealthyDeviant.com) is a collection of tools and tactics you can use for the rest of your life, if you like. Some of these tools are specifically designed to help you chart your experience and maintain momentum as you go through the Healthy Deviant Adventure program. But you can use them whenever, however, and for as long as you choose.

There are also a number of additional resources that I think you'll find helpful as you move forward in your own Healthy Deviant explorations—not just now, but well into the future. And, of course, I am here, too. Please consider me part of your toolkit. You can find me on my social channels, through my websites (HealthyDeviant.com and PilarGerasimo.com), and at some point, I'd love to see you at one of my workshops, talks, retreats, or other live events. In the meantime, delve as deep as you like into these goodies. Oh, and then please read part 5, if you're feeling it! (In some ways, it's the most important part of this book.)

Daily Deviance Journal Pages

Interactive field notes for each day of the program. You can find blanks at the back of this chapter and you can find a downloadable workbook containing titled Journal Pages for each of the fourteen days of the program at HealthyDeviant.com/toolkit.

Healthy Deviant Adventure Tracker

Check-off chart with overviews of each day. You can use this instead of or in addition to the Daily Deviance Journal Pages. Totally up to you. There's a blank at the back of this chapter, and there's a larger, two-page version available at HealthyDeviant.com/toolkit.

Healthy Deviant Signage

I've created some post-able reminders (including a "Healthy Deviant Adventure in Progress" sign) you can stick to your fridge, car dashboard, and bathroom mirror, plus some top-secret signage and talismans that only fellow Healthy Deviants will recognize. Again, you'll find some of these at the back of this chapter, and you'll find more at HealthyDeviant.com /toolkit. And of course, you can make your own (a fun Morning Minutes or Ultradian Rhythm Break project!).

When You're Freaking Out

It is the nature of Healthy Deviance to put you up against all kinds of conventional forces and institutionalized barriers (as well as insidious saboteurs) that will make you feel like you've lost your mind or have taken on more than you can possibly handle. For those moments, here are just a few revolutionary resources to help you reclaim your sanity and center:

Healthy Deviant E-Toolkit

In addition to all the Daily Deviance Journal Pages and Healthy Deviant Adventure Tracker, this downloadable e-book also contains some bonus material that wouldn't quite fit into this printed book or that I thought to include after it went to press. It provides links to some guided meditations and other resources you might enjoy on those days when it seems the whole world has gone mad, when it's all just too hard, or when you just don't feel like doing whatever else you're supposed to be doing right now. Find all these goodies at HealthyDeviant.com/toolkit.

RevolutionaryAct.com and the "101 Revolutionary Ways to Be Healthy" Mobile App

A repository of Healthy Deviant wisdom I created in partnership with *Experience Life* magazine and Life Time—The Healthy Way of Life Company. Both the site and the app feature the "101 Revolutionary Ways to Be Healthy" (a thought-provoking, interactive infographic inspired by my *Manifesto for Thriving in a Mixed-Up World*), but the app includes links to deeper reading from *Experience Life* on each of the 101 topics. Thanks to the generosity of *Experience Life* and Life Time, I'm in the process of integrating Revolutionary Act with my new Healthy Deviant work, so you can expect to see this collection morph and evolve over the next year or so. Even kids enjoy the 101 Ways, so if you haven't checked them out, please do. More at RevolutionaryAct.com, or find the app in your favorite app store.

Being Healthy Is a Revolutionary Act: A Manifesto for Thriving in a Mixed-Up World

This is the manifesto that started it all—my early thinking on Healthy Deviance, before I'd given it that name. This chapbook is available as a free download and also as a limited edition print chapbook (along with other Healthy Deviant swag) through the store at HealthyDeviant.com.

My "Revolutionary Acts" Column

Between 2013 and 2016, I wrote up thirty-seven of the 101 Revolutionary Ways to Be Healthy as a "Revolutionary Acts" column for *Experience Life* magazine. It also appeared as a long-running blog for *Huffington Post*. I'm proud that this series won a gold FOLIO award from the American Society of

Magazine Editors. Someday, I'm thinking I'll turn them into a book of their own, but for now you can find them (along with a bunch of my other writing for *Experience Life*) at ExperienceLife .com/author/pgerasimo.

The Living Experiment Podcast

This is the podcast I co-host with Dallas Hartwig. Our motto is "rethink your choices, reclaim your life." We've recorded more than a hundred episodes so far (covering everything from imposter syndrome to poop, plus two separate episodes on Healthy Deviance), and I hope we'll be doing more soon. A lot of listeners have written to say the podcast changed their lives in some way. I suspect what happened is that they listened and then *decided to change their lives,* but why split hairs? More at LivingExperiment .com, or find it on your favorite podcast platform. Definitely listen to the "Morning," "Pause," and "Sleep" episodes, because they loosely map to the Renegade Rituals.

Experience Life Magazine

This is the whole-person healthy living magazine I created back in 2001 in partnership with Life Time—the Healthy Way of Life Company. It's been going strong, in print, for nearly twenty years now and is still run by a team of terrific journalists who know how to separate trash from treasure, and how to cover the topics that really matter to health seekers and Healthy Deviants of all stripes—from nutrition and movement to mental-emotional health and socio-cultural issues. Making this magazine certainly changed *my* life, and I'm proud that it still covers a lot of important subjects that other health magazines don't. Here are just a few articles I'd encourage you to consider reading (you can locate them by typing their titles into the search box at ExperienceLife.com, or find links in the online toolkit at HealthyDeviant.com/toolkit:

- **"Stages of Change"** Break a habit. Achieve a goal. Transform your life. It all starts with assessing your readiness to change.

- **"Weight Loss Rules to Rethink"** Forget what you've been told. Forget what you think you know. Forget the old rules—and you might just start making some headway.

- **"Easier by the Day: 9 Ways Exercise Gets Less Difficult as You Go"** Wanna know a little secret about exercise? It gets easier, more fun, and more rewarding with each passing day.

- **"The Healing Power of Sleep"** New science shows that sleep is essential to our mental and physical health—and most of us aren't getting enough.

- **"A Real Pleasure"** When it comes to creating the conditions for optimal health, we know that managing stress is important. But it turns out that dealing with our anxieties and negative emotional reactions is only half the battle. Discover why an ample supply of enjoyable, positive experiences is equally essential to your well-being—and how you can go about giving life's pleasures the healthy emphasis they deserve.

- **"Take a Break"** Random moments of unproductive time don't just make you healthier, happier, and more resilient. They help you work smarter, too.

- **"The Whole Thing"** Enriched this, supplemental that. Look behind the hype and you'll discover that whole foods deliver nutrition that fragmented and isolated nutrients simply can't beat.

- **"Gluten: The Whole Story"** Gluten troubles were once thought to be a problem primarily for those with celiac disease. But recent research indicates that gluten-related disorders extend to a far broader population and affect far more than the digestive system.

- **"Autoimmune Disorders: When Your Body Turns on You"** There's been a stark rise in autoimmune disorders over the past fifty years, from type 1 diabetes and multiple sclerosis to celiac disease and asthma. The first step toward a cure is understanding and controlling the causes.

- **"How to Heal a Leaky Gut"** Your intestines are home to a great deal of your digestive system, nervous system, and immune system. Here's how to keep them healthy and avoid leaky gut syndrome.

Refine Your Life Workbook

I created this collection of interactive personal-development exercises as a sort of self-coaching "greatest hits" collection back in the late 1990s, because I couldn't afford a life coach at the time, and I couldn't find all the stuff I wanted and needed in one place. The workbook covers values, vision, goals, and action planning, and it includes both proven coaching tools (like a Life Wheel), as well as some original ones (like my Goal Flower exercise). It also features some selected reading from *Experience Life* magazine. You can find a downloadable version at HealthyDeviant.com.

"Your Ideal Day" Visualization

I've been blown away by how many requests I've had from therapists who want to use this guided meditation with their clients, and I still use it myself on a regular basis. The MP3 collection (originally created in partnership with my pal Brian Johnson's En*theos initiative) includes an introduction, the meditation, and some affirmation tracks set over binaural beats (that's fancy language for "inaudible brain-optimizing sounds"). You can find a link to the free MP3 download at PilarGerasimo.com/resources.

Optimize with Brian Johnson

My genius friend Brian Johnson has been collecting and distilling life-changing wisdom for decades now, and he's just the best at it, period. Check out his Philosophers Notes, Optimal Living 101 courses and +1 videos, Optimize with Brian Johnson podcast, Optimize Coach programs, community, and more, all at Optimize.me.

Signs of Success

Not sure that any of this is making any difference at all? Still waiting for the scale to budge or for your pants to fit looser? Stop waiting! Instead, use this handy top-ten list (you *knew* there had to one, right?) to tune into some of the most frequently overlooked indicators of real progress:

10. Your eyes look just a little bit clearer and like "your lights are back on."

9. Conventional magazine covers and television ads start seeming utterly ridiculous to you.

8. You start enjoying your Morning Minutes so much that you decide to extend them well beyond three minutes.

7. One day, you notice that you are fatigued, distracted, grumpy, or hungry, and instead of getting down on yourself, you think, "Hey, I bet I need an Ultradian Rhythm Break!"

6. You go on a walk and leave your phone behind; you then start wishing everybody else did too. Bonus points: You subtly try out one or more of the Three Walks while you are walking, just for fun.

5. You practice some small act of self-care or self-kindness, and rather than seeing it as an act of self-indulgence, you see it as an act of Healthy Deviant defiance.

4. You notice you have to go to the bathroom, and you respond to that call without delay.

3. You notice you are thirsty and immediately go get some water.

2. One day, you feel just a tiny bit more hopeful or more energetic, and think, "Hmm, maybe this weird Healthy Deviant Adventure approach is actually working! "

1. You start looking around for the other Healthy Deviants in your midst, thinking, "I know I can't be the only one … " And suddenly, you start seeing them everywhere.

THE TOOLS

- Daily Deviance Journal Pages
- Healthy Deviant Adventure Trackers
- Healthy Deviant Signage

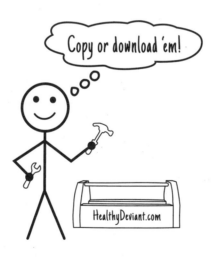

Copy or download 'em!

HealthyDeviant.com

Date: _____

Renegade Rituals

Morning Minutes

Desire/willingness to do?   Yes / No
Done?   Yes / No

If yes, nice!
  Chosen activity?   _____
  How long?   3 min. / other: _____
  Enjoyed?   Yes / No

If no, hmm, interesting.
  What got in the way? (other people, environment, me, etc.)
  _____

Daily Reading? Yes / No   Any reflections?

AM Ultradian Rhythm Break

Desire/willingness to do?   Yes / No
Done?   Yes / No

If done, nice!
  Chosen activity?   _____
  How long?   10   15   20 min./ other: ____
  Noticeable result? Yes / No

If not done, hmm, interesting.
  What got in the way? (other people, environment, me, etc.)
  _____

PM Ultradian Rhythm Break

Desire/willingness to do?   Yes / No
Done?   Yes / No

If done, nice!
  Chosen activity?   _____
  How long?   10   15   20 min./ other: _____
  Noticeable result? Yes / No

If not done, hmm, interesting.
  What got in the way? (other people, environment, me, etc.)
  _____

Nighttime Wind-Down

Desire/willingness to do?   Yes / No
Done?   Yes / No

If yes, nice!
  How long?   5   10   15   20 min./ other: ____
  Enjoyed?   Yes / No

If no, hmm, interesting.
  What got in the way? (other people, environment, me, etc.)

○ All screens off
○ Turn-down of lights, volume, pace, intensity, temp
○ Puttery clean-up and next-day prep
○ Warm water/herbal tea
○ Evening Ablutions

_____

© Pilar Gerasimo 2020   →

continued ...

Check-In

What was the condition of my body-mind for most of today?

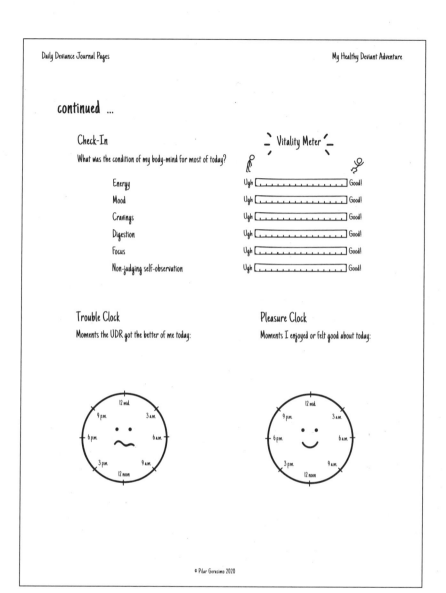

Energy

Mood

Cravings

Digestion

Focus

Non-judging self-observation

Vitality Meter

Ugh [   ] Good!

Ugh [   ] Good!

Ugh [   ] Good!

Ugh [   ] Good!

Ugh [   ] Good!

Ugh [   ] Good!

Trouble Clock

Moments the UDR got the better of me today:

Pleasure Clock

Moments I enjoyed or felt good about today:

© Pilar Gerasimo 2020

For full-size versions, visit HealthyDeviant.com.

Healthy Deviant Adventure Tracker: Phase 1

~ Renegade Rituals ~

- Vitality Meter -

	Morning Minutes	URB #1	URB #2	Nighttime Wind-Down		
Day 1: Start Where You Are	☐	☐	☐	☐	Low — High
Day 2: Gather Courage	☐	☐	☐	☐	Low — High
Day 3: Find Things Right	☐	☐	☐	☐	Low — High
Day 4: Cultivate Willingess	☐	☐	☐	☐	Low — High
Day 5: Call BS	☐	☐	☐	☐	Low — High
Day 6: Ask for What You Want	☐	☐	☐	☐	Low — High
Day 7: Celebrate Small Successes	☐	☐	☐	☐	Low — High

© Pilar Gerasimo 2020

Healthy Deviant Adventure Tracker: Phase 2

Renegade Rituals

	Morning Minutes	URB #1	URB #2	Nighttime Wind-Down	Vitality Meter
Day 8: Abandon Victim Thinking	☐	☐	☐	☐	Low — High
Day 9: Find Your Edge	☐	☐	☐	☐	Low — High
Day 10: Renegotiate Reality	☐	☐	☐	☐	Low — High
Day 11: Act As If	☐	☐	☐	☐	Low — High
Day 12: Stake Your Claim	☐	☐	☐	☐	Low — High
Day 13: Expand Your Horizon	☐	☐	☐	☐	Low — High
Day 14: Bask, Beware, Repeat	☐	☐	☐	☐	Low — High

© Pilar Gerasimo 2020

For full-size versions, visit HealthyDeviant.com.

Cut out and fold for tent cards.

HEALTHY 😉 DEVIANT®

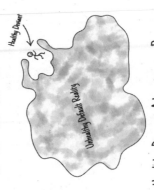

Healthy Deviant Adventure in Progress

Cut out and fold for tent card. ↘

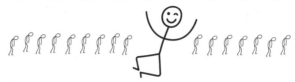

Break the Rules ...

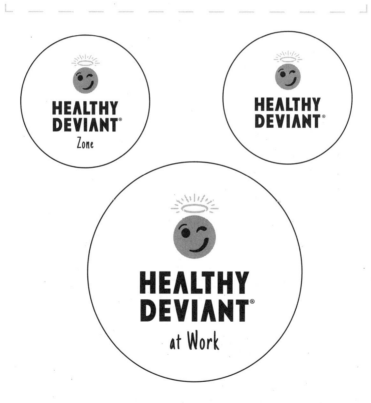

HEALTHY
DEVIANT®
Zone

HEALTHY
DEVIANT®

HEALTHY
DEVIANT®
at Work

Cut out and hole punch for hang tags.
Get color versions of all these signs at HealthyDeviant.com.

Cut out and fold for tent cards.

Nighttime Wind-Down Begins at: _____

Is It Time for a U.R.B. Yet?

Later Please, Morning Minutes in Progress

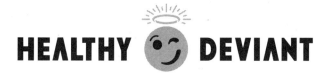

HEALTHY DEVIANT

Get ready for weirdness.
Then check off each day of your Healthy Deviant Adventure as you go ...

Week 1
Start Where You Are

| 1 | 2 | 3 | 4 | 5 | 6 | 7 |

Week 2
Raise Your Game

| 1 | 2 | 3 | 4 | 5 | 6 | 7 |

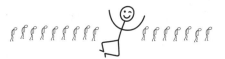

© Pilar Gerasimo 2020

For full-size versions, visit HealthyDeviant.com.

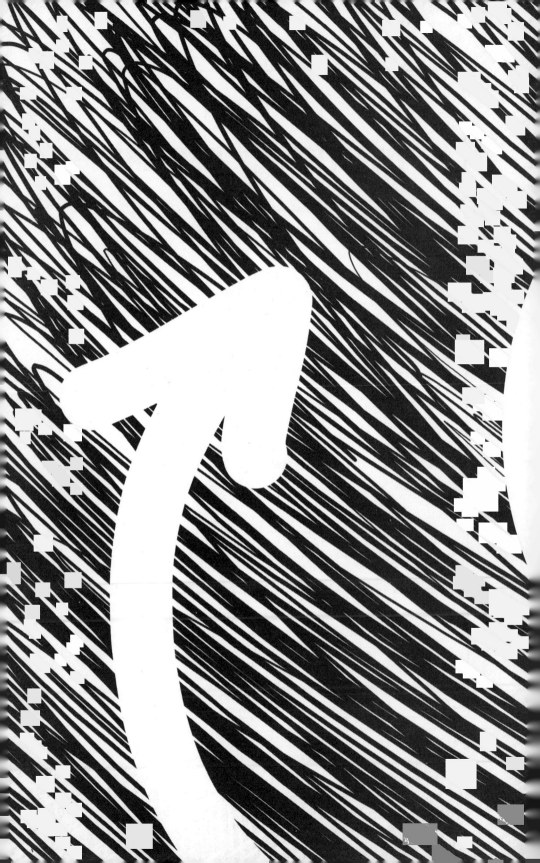

PART 5

Taking It to the Streets

This hour in history needs a dedicated circle
of transformed nonconformists....
The saving of our world from pending doom will come,
not through the complacent adjustment
of the conforming majority, but through the
creative maladjustment of a non-conforming minority....
Human salvation lies in the hands
of the creatively maladjusted.

—MARTIN LUTHER KING JR.

The Healthy Deviant Manifesto

It is not because things are difficult that we do not dare.
It is because we do not dare that they are difficult.

—SENECA

It is possible to opt out of the sick status quo and begin creating a better world. Just know that if you choose to do what it takes to be healthy and thriving in our current crazy-unhealthy world, you are quickly going to join the ranks of a small but powerful minority. You will, as noted, become something of an anomaly. You have to get comfortable with that, take pride in it, and, on some level, make it a part of your identity.

To become one of the healthy-happy few, you'll need to develop the capacity to go against established norms, and to quickly recognize when the forces of our unhealthy society are messing with your mind and body. You'll need to begin to take pleasure in your Healthy Deviance and find strength in the knowledge that you are refusing to be assimilated. You'll need to repeatedly wake up and remember that you've got better things to do with your life energy than having it sucked into the conventional vortex of doom.

Is any of this easy or convenient? Not at first, but it gets easier as you go, and particularly as you find other renegades like you. With time and practice, it actually turns out to be pretty fun. It is certainly much easier than being chronically ill and miserable.

From time to time, I still get bogged down by the difficulties and ugliness of the world we're living in. I fall off my own healthy bandwagon and find myself moping around, feeling depleted and oppressed by The Man. When that happens, I find it helps to have a few, simple imperatives to follow.

With that in mind, I present you with...

The Healthy Deviant Manifesto

1. Subvert the Unhealthy Default Reality.

Dare to make disruptive healthy choices daily—even (or especially) in the face of resistance. Ask for what you want. Stand up for your health-preserving rights and preferences. Keep your wits about you, and refuse to let the dominant-culture machine roll over your healthy autonomy.

2. Call out the crazy.

Point to our society's unhealthy madness so others can start seeing it, too. Speak up for the healthy truths you hold to be self-evident. Laugh in the face of nonsense, even when it's official, authoritative nonsense. When you see body shaming, bad advice, or unrealistic "aspirational" imagery you think is daft, say so. Wave your fist Roll your eyes. Let off steam. Then get back to your own Healthy Deviant business.

3. Make it a party.

Welcome, support, and seek common ground with health seekers of all stripes. Seek and form Healthy Deviant communities. See healthy living as an opportunity for growth, discovery, and self-expression, not a grim battle or competition. Enjoy the process. Make healthy living a fun, celebratory, open-hearted, inclusive gathering that everybody wants to join.

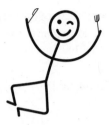

* * *

Wait, that's it? No diet, no exercise, no call for widespread action or a zillion-dollar investment from private-public partnerships? That is correct.

The Problem with Grandiose, Zillion-Dollar Solutions

Here's the thing about all those huge programs that get announced with fanfare, decorated with star-studded sponsors, and funded by taxpayer money: They accomplish almost nothing. Instead, they tend to *mis-define* the problem and offer ineffective solutions. Typically, those solutions serve to increase the power and wealth of some already powerful and wealthy industries, like the processed-food industry, weight-loss industry, pharmaceutical or health-care industry.

Consider, for example, the "Wellness Moonshot" announced by the Global Wellness Institute at the Davos World Economic Forum in 2017. Featuring the usual panoply of celebrity health experts—some of whom have long delivered the same ineffective, oversimplified, or just plain wrong-headed advice that got us here in the first place—the Wellness Moonshot has a grand goal: "Preventing chronic disease."

That sounds good, at least on the surface. But the entire thrust of the messaging from this Moonshot subtly implies that once you *have* a chronic disease, your wellness is a lost cause. And that's not true. As proven by Dr. Terry Wahls, Dr. David Perlmutter, Dr. Dale Bredesen, Dr. Rangan Chatterjee, Dr. Mark Hyman, and others, many chronic diseases can be *reversed.* But that message isn't getting out there via big, industry-led efforts like the Global Wellness Institute, and it probably never will.

Here's why: The Wellness Moonshot focuses primarily on industry as a solution (seeing global illness as a business opportunity, naturally). It doesn't openly acknowledge the systemic reasons (including industrial influences and incentives) that so many people are inclined to get many chronic diseases in the first place.

The high-minded blather associated with this kind of program, even when well intended, almost always comes down to the tropes of personal responsibility and prescribed "healthy choices."

And often those are choices that prove near impossible or, worse, totally counterproductive.

We can't prevent chronic disease by scaling and underwriting (even to "moonshot" proportions) the very solutions that have helped to create them. That's what USDA nutrition guidelines and MyPlate.gov have done. It's what the Diabetes Prevention Program and "Look Ahead" initiatives have done. It's what a lot of the advice from American Dietetic Association, American Heart Association, and American Cancer Society have done, and it looks pretty much like what Wellness Moonshot might be aimed to do.

Solutions that suggest warmed-over strategies of just eating less and exercising more, counting calories, reducing fat, eating more whole grains (meaning flours, starches, and sugars), relying on willpower, getting more medical screenings, taking more pharmaceutical drugs, and so on, simply *do not work.* At least, they do not work in the context of the society we are living in now.

So, this is what I'm proposing. We figure it out and we do it together. In our own homes, our own workplaces, our own schools, our own communities. We advocate for and empower each other. We point out that *we are the bright spots,* and following our example is going to work a whole lot better than all the grandiose, top-down, zillion-dollar solutions that haven't worked at all.

If you are a parent, decide that you are going to raise a bunch of Healthy Deviants, knowing that they will undoubtedly rebel, suffer the consequences, and, at some point, come back around to say they really should have listened to you more. According to my mother, this will be extremely gratifying.

If you are an executive or business owner, don't spend a million dollars hiring some corporate wellness consultancy that tells you to put carrot sticks in the break room. Instead, canvass the healthiest people in your organization to find out what *they* are doing and how you could make it easier for others to follow suit.

If you are a public-policy person, stop taking your advice from industry insiders. Decide to get legitimately healthy yourself, and talk to other legitimately healthy people (*not* just celebrities and rich people) who actually seem to be having a dramatic, positive effect on the lives of others.

Use this logic to figure out how you can be part of the solution, how you can *live* the Healthy Deviant Manifesto wherever you happen to live, work, love, and play. In this way, we can cease fighting the current reality, and in R. Buckminster Fuller's wise words "build a new model that makes the existing model obsolete."

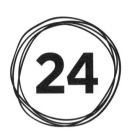

Deviant Disruption

A CASE FOR CIVILIZED DISOBEDIENCE

Disobedience, in the eyes of anyone who has read history, is man's original virtue. It is through disobedience that progress has been made, through disobedience and through rebellion.

—OSCAR WILDE

Now you know what most people don't. If you've been reading this book or doing any part of the Healthy Deviant Adventure program, you are *doing things* most people don't. And if you've gotten some return for that, some new sense of energy or possibility or potential, you have entered into a domain that most people never enter.

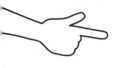

You are, at least in some way, a Healthy Deviant.

Now, where do you go with that? You could keep it to yourself. You could spend years quietly "perfecting" your Healthy Deviant game. Or you could begin sharing what you know with others. You could begin holding open the small tear you created in the Unhealthy Default Reality's membrane, and inviting other people to join you on the outside.

There's a reason the final call of the Healthy Deviant Manifesto is "make it a party." We cannot vanquish the Unhealthy Default Reality on our own. We need a boots-on-the-ground movement of Healthy Deviants all pulling for each other and helping to pull their loved ones and community members free from the Unhealthy Default Reality ooze.

What does this look like? It looks like all the little changes you make to your home and office environment, all the little accommodations you request everywhere you go, all the little licenses you take in the service of making things easier for all health seekers (remember: It's better to ask for forgiveness than permission).

It looks like conspiring, forming committees, assembling task forces, and building petitions focused on getting higher-ups to get behind your Healthy Deviant efforts, convincing them to underwrite and amplify them for reasons (reduced cost, improved outcomes) that matter to them.

It looks like strategic disruption at work and at school, a call for the accommodation of *real* healthy choices and health-producing patterns wherever we spend our time. It looks like a rejection of the status quo, always-on mass media, and all of the unrealistic ideals, distractions, and stressors it proffers.

It looks like a radical redesign of conventional medicine, and a takeover of so-called "preventative" health strategies that are actually feeder mechanisms for dead-end treatments and setups for distress and disease. I'm guessing a lot of fed-up, functionally trained practitioners and health coaches will wind up leading this charge.

It also looks like advocacy and organizing at the policy level. It looks like supporting the system-wide changes that empower people to take good, empowered care of themselves rather than deepening their dependency on a broken medical model and incentivizing their purchases of commodity-based junk foods. It looks like true health education in our schools and a shifting of the unhealthy products and propaganda that surround our children. It may well involve marching in the streets—not necessarily for Healthy Deviance, per se, but for all the rights, choices, and freedoms that make up its foundations.

Redefining Nonviolence

A few years back, Mark Hyman, MD, told me about a conversation he'd had over lunch with Reverend Bernice King, daughter of Dr. Martin Luther King Jr. and head of the Martin Luther King Center for Nonviolent Social Change. He told me that it sounded like the Center was considering expanding their definition of *nonviolence* to expressly include the avoidance of mental, emotional, and physical damage brought on by obesity and chronic illness.

I inquired with the King Center archives and dug around online, and while I have not been able to find any record of that expanded definition having been officially adopted, it certainly seems consistent with the King Center's values and its "Nonviolence 365" initiative. And if a broader definition like that ever *were* officially adopted, it would appropriately reflect the fact that one of the most pernicious forms of social oppression now occurs in the form of lifestyle-driven chronic illnesses—illnesses experienced at disproportionally high rates among people of color. It would acknowledge that institutionalized health disparities pose significant threats not just to individuals but also to our society as a whole.

I have now come to expand my own definition of nonviolence to encompass violence against one's own body-mind. I've also come to understand "violence" as inclusive of the longterm pain and damage done to others by institutional, financial, or political means. I'm clear that while cultivating Healthy Deviance can produce positive and transformative results for anyone, it holds both particular promise and particular challenge for any person or community struggling under socially oppressive burdens (including racial discrimination and economic injustice) that predispose them to compromised health and vitality.

So, how can we make this a less violent, damaging, and harmful world for all? I think it starts with accepting that disruption is necessary and in all our best interests. And that it requires not just intention, but effort, investment, and endurance. It requires looking beyond disease statistics and population-health priorities toward real, lifelong health-creation for all.

Finding Meaning in
Creative Maladjustment

If there ever *is* a march for Healthy Deviance, I hope to be on the front lines, waving my Healthy Deviant banner. And I hope there are millions of people just like you marching right along beside me. But even if we don't have a formal march, it's important to recognize that most of us Healthy Deviants are demonstrating, protesting, and resisting being assimilated every day of our lives. That's a good thing, as long as we don't run ourselves ragged or numb. Because the Unhealthy Default Reality runs on our apathy, passivity, and victimization. Just as it is fueled by our illness, our depression, our feelings of *less-than-itis*.

We cannot allow the Unhealthy Default Reality to define what a healthy body or healthy life looks like, because to the Unhealthy Default Reality, "healthy" is a just another way to suck us in. It's another way to get us to buy what we don't need, to chase what works against us, and to participate in reinforcing the systems that tear us down.

Instead, let us keep in mind the words of Dr. Martin Luther King Jr., who so eloquently drew the world's attention not just to the injustices of racial and ethnic oppression but also to the wrongness and waste of *all* oppressive, needlessly constraining ideas of who—and how—we should be.

In September 1967, just seven months before he was assassinated, Dr. Martin Luther King delivered a lecture to the American Psychological Association titled "The Role of the Behavioral Scientist in the Civil Rights Movement." In it, he addressed the important role social scientists had to play in fostering what he called "creative maladjustment"—the willingness to challenge destructive social norms and institutional constructs in favor of a more just, ethical, and promising reality.

In his talk, Dr. King asserted that "there are some things in our society, some things in our world, to which we should never be adjusted. There are some things concerning which we must always be maladjusted if we are to be people of good will." King then called for the creation of a new organization, an "International Association for the Advancement of Creative Maladjustment," arguing that the prophet Amos, Abraham Lincoln, and Thomas Jefferson were good examples of admirably "maladjusted" individuals and that we might all benefit from following their example in questioning the troubling conventions of our time. "Through such creative maladjustment," Dr. King wrote, "we may be able to emerge from the bleak and desolate midnight of man's inhumanity to man, into the bright and glittering daybreak of freedom and justice."[47]

The version of reality in which most of us are living runs on just that sort of inhumanity. It robs us of our dignity and autonomy. It siphons our energy and resources, keeping us captive in hamster wheels where our efforts generate only more power for the grid that keeps the Unhealthy Default Reality's engines operating at full throttle.

It's time for us to take that power back. It's time for us to see our health as something more than a stock-image ideal, the absence of disease, or a "normal" set of lab values. It's time for us to remember that health is our first human freedom, and to reclaim it as our birthright.

Health is both our passport to a better way of living and a get-out-of-jail-free card—a license to practice living in the ways that bring out the best not just in us but also in all the parts of this world that we influence and touch.

Let us begin practicing now.

In *Let Us Now Praise Famous Men,* James Agee wrote: " 'Adjustment' to a sick and insane environment is of itself not 'health' but sickness and insanity." That is so true, and it sounds a lot like that Jiddu Krishnamurti quote I shared at this book's outset: "It is no measure of health to be well-adjusted to a profoundly sick society." These quotes, and many of the other quotes I've shared in these pages, run through my mind on a daily basis. They keep me feeling sane in what often seems like a crazy, mixed-up world.

The thing is, though, even when you know this stuff, even when you hold it in your heart and feel it in your bones, being maladjusted to one's society is still no walk in the park. And if you have somehow made it to part 5 of this book, I am guessing you know that from experience. As one of this world's "creatively maladjusted" types, you have likely felt both the rewards and the costs of your creativity.

As you explore the realms of Healthy Deviance, you'll find that deviating from socially accepted norms and patterns, even in ways as innocuous as I've offered here, can and does disrupt the status quo. It can invite teasing or pushback—particularly from people who haven't committed to taking care of themselves in the ways you've chosen to, or who subscribe to more conventional notions of what "healthcare" looks like.

At times, that can feel discouraging. Happily, shaking things up can also feel profoundly energizing and exciting. And in the long run, the rewards of being a Healthy Deviant vastly outweigh the costs. Initially, though, it can require a certain kind of damn-the-torpedoes determination—one that only a small number of bright-spot outliers are currently managing to sustain.

You can be one of those healthy, bright-spot outliers, if you choose. And it really doesn't have to be all that difficult or uncomfortable. Embracing the perspectives and strategies I've shared here will definitely make it easier.

The bigger promise of Healthy Deviance, though, lies in making the process of outwitting the Unhealthy Default Reality more fun, meaningful, appealing, and rewarding. That's important, because if we want to live in a healthier, happier world, we need a whole lot more of us to start taking better care of ourselves and each other.

If enough Healthy Deviants start waking up and extracting themselves from the Unhealthy Default Reality, we can begin creating that healthier, happier world now. You could help make it happen. Maybe you already are.

Take It Easy, Take It Slow

Not sure you're ready to become a Healthy Deviant? Too overwhelmed by your own pressing challenges to get excited about changing the world? That's okay. Just start by taking a closer look at how the Unhealthy Default Reality might be affecting you. Look at how you could start judging and blaming yourself a bit less and supporting yourself a bit more.

Little by little, you'll find yourself discovering your own winding paths into Amplified Awareness, Preemptive Repair, and Continuous Growth and Learning. You'll start tinkering with your own Renegade Rituals and tailoring them to your personal needs and preferences.

At that point, you'll have embarked on a Healthy Deviant journey of your own making. Which is, come to think of it, pretty much the only kind of Healthy Deviant journey there is.

EPILOGUE

A Bizarrely Better World

We sense that "normal" isn't coming back,
that we are being born into a new normal:
a new kind of society, a new relationship to the earth,
a new experience of being human.

—CHARLES EISENSTEIN

Imagine, if you will, a world in which the current ratio of healthy to unhealthy people was inverted. What if, instead of most people struggling and only a tiny minority thriving, it was the other way around?

Envision, just for a moment, what it would be like to live and work in a world where most people were in reasonably good shape most of the time. Imagine a society where homes, schools, workplaces, and cities were designed by healthy people with healthy preferences in mind, where health-supporting priorities and policies were supported, and where chronic illness was rare.

What would it be like to live in a world where most people were healthy and happy most of the time? With that many well-nourished, well-rested people and that much energy, capacity, and resilience on tap, imagine the challenges we could solve. Imagine the suffering and injustices we could relieve, and waste we could spare, the resources we could unleash, the beauty and bounty we could create.

What would it be like if the super-healthy majority were able to easily help care for, encourage, and support those for whom good health, by virtue of some misfortune, was presently out of reach? If the vast majority of us were strong, centered, vital, and aware, and if we had patience, energy, and creativity to spare, what kind of world would we design and cocreate?

If the Unhealthy Default Reality were no more, and the Healthy Default Reality were to take its place, how would our preferences for healthy patterns, products, and services change? How would those preferences change our economy, our society, our daily lives? What would our communities, schools, and built environments be like? What would we teach our children, and what un-truths would we cease trying to cram down their throats?

How would health care evolve? How about agriculture and the energy industry? How would we invest our money and our time? Who would we put in charge of corporations and civic institutions? Who would decide to run for and get elected to public office? Would we even need prisons and a "corrections" system anymore?

Let's take it a wild and crazy step further.

What if the *whole world* was aligned around healthy priorities and preferences, and was aware that the health of one nation depended directly on the health of all the others. How might we behave? How would we treat each other? What entrenched, global problems might we solve? What destructive, short-sighted efforts might we cease? What wasted resources might we be able to conserve, regenerate, and redirect? What kind of future might we begin embracing for ourselves and our planet?

I don't have the answers to all those questions, but I think it is fair to assume that a world formed by the preferences and priorities of healthy, happy people—people who are clear that our health and happiness is interconnected—would be a vastly better, more beautiful, and harmonious place to live. So why not go about building that world now, person by person, family by family, workplace by workplace, community by community?

Here, in my Healthy Deviant heart and soul, is what I know to be true:

- By consciously forging super-resilient, Healthy Deviant identities, we can empower others and help change the world for the better.

- By challenging counterproductive conventions and modeling more successful approaches, we can become a growing throng of bright-spot outliers who advance healthier new norms.

- By reframing our challenges, by rejecting doomed dominant-culture tactics in favor of more innovative and effective strategies, we can blaze more rewarding paths toward authentic health and happiness.

Look, none of us needs to fix all the world's ills all on our own. But we could, right now, wake from the stupor of the Unhealthy Default Reality and begin considering the exhilarating promise of making our vision for a healthier world a reality. One Healthy Deviant person, family, and community at a time, we could do that. We'd be crazy not to.

ACKNOWLEDGMENTS

It turns out what you need to be a successful Healthy Deviant is the same stuff you need to complete a big, challenging project like writing a book (particularly a category-defying, unconventional book that took five years to write). That includes determination, willingness to experiment, a certain amount of crazy, and the support of a whole lot of good people.

This particular book would not have been possible without the help of a bunch of extraordinary folks who contributed at every stage of the process and who taught me virtually everything I know. I stand on the shoulders of some very talented giants, and I cannot possibly name them all. My sincere appreciation goes out to each of them, though, with a special thanks to the following.

My agent, Scott Edelstein, for coming out of retirement to take me on as a client and then walking me through the long, largely uncharted, and often maddening process of making my unwieldy collection of materials into a bona fide book.

Agents Joy Tutela and Richard Pine, for investing time and energy, very early on, in helping me get clearer about what this book did and did not want to be.

Alison Knowles, Susan Bumps, Bevin Donahue, Ebonie Ledbetter, and the whole team at North Atlantic Books for seeing the potential in this book from the start, for being willing to embrace my highly collaborative tendencies, and for not insisting on making this book too "normal."

Lisa Braun Dubbels of Catalyst Publicity for helping to get the word out.

Dara Moskowitz Grumdahl, at whose kitchen table this book was revived after a close brush with death, for hours of insight-provoking walks and talks and meals, for timely texts, and for generous wine-pouring from start to finish.

My friend and podcasting partner Dallas Hartwig for endless conversations and collaborations, for helping me workshop much of this material on

The Living Experiment podcast, and for not letting me quit halfway through.

My soul brother Brian Johnson, founder and Chief Philosopher of Optimize Enterprises, with whom I've swapped ideas, insights, enthusiasms, great books, and better-world visions for nearly two decades now. Bri, deep bow. *Let's do this.*

Geneen Roth for all kinds of inspiration and wisdom, for luminous truth-telling (if you haven't read her most recent book, *This Messy Magnificent Life,* please do), and for the long-distance daily meditation experiment that gave me the mental space and equanimity to finish the book with much more ease than I began it.

Betsy Lane for editorial support both with the proposal and the manuscript. I'm not sure I would have finished the proposal without you, Bets.

Lydia Anderson, creative director at *Experience Life,* for more than a decade of creative collaboration and friendship. Years ago, as a personal favor, Lydia (a brilliant fine artist and designer) drew some of the first stick-figure and line drawings for my *Refine Your Life* workbook, including the base drawing for the "landscape of personal change" illustration in chapter 19. The simplicity and charm of Lydia's drawings inspired the ones I subsequently created for this book—a project I would never have undertaken without her encouragement.

Jamie Martin, editor-in-chief, along with the entire *Experience Life* magazine team, for cocreating the magazine, for giving me the space to do what I love for oh-so-many years now, and for running the first illustrated feature on Healthy Deviance ever printed in a national periodical.

Life Time, *Experience Life*'s parent company, for green-lighting the project when it was still just an experimental, very expensive idea and for continuing to support my work in so many ways ever since. The magazine now reaches three million people with each issue? Wow. That still gets me.

Brittany Play-Button for her talent and skill in helping me evolve a number of my first, chicken-scratch illustration and infograph efforts into far more presentable and comprehensible versions of themselves, and for guiding me through the confusing world of digital illustration software tools.

Rebecca Kilde for invaluable help in framing up an early version of the "Ape in the Arcade" drawing, which otherwise would have been well beyond my perspective-drawing capabilities.

Tim Tate for thoughtful indexing, input, and last-minute typo catches. Adam Hadhazy for early research and fact-checking assistance.

Art director/designer Brian Johnson (another Brian Johnson!) of Box 86, LLC, for jumping into a big, complex book-design project with fearless creativity, admirable endurance, and the *best* collaborative problem-solving talents imaginable.

Penny and Bill George for years of encouragement and support, and for setting an example of what it looks like to be invested in healing at scale.

Dorothy Kalins, my longtime mentor and friend, for seeing the potential in my rudimentary editorial work, for sticking with me through thick and thin, and for providing wise, gracious guidance every step of the way.

Cat Thompson, Martha Ross Parker, Bill Hillsman, Tom Weise, Nate Garvis, Dan Buettner, Chip Heath, Kris Carr, Kate Larsen, Martia Nelson, Marilyn Moohr, Lana Holmes, Maureen Pelton, Tony Schwartz, and countless other mentors, teachers, authors, coaches, and friends (including many at Mills College, the Stanford and Yale Publishing Courses, and Lafayette Morehouse) who nudged, encouraged, and helped me along at a thousand different intervals.

Cindy Joseph, one of my dearest friends and coconspirators, who left this earthly plane on the same day I submitted my final book proposal, for her years of inspiration, urging, and enthusiastic cheerleading, for lending the pro-age movement voice and heart, and for so beautifully modeling what it looks like to be a radiant, happy, silver-haired, self-realized woman who is dancing to the beat of her own drum and following her dreams.

Drs. Mark Hyman, David Ludwig, Jeffrey Bland, Michael Stone, Frank Lipman, David Perlmutter, Terry Wahls, Deanna Minich, Tom O'Bryan, and so many others for introducing me to smart, progressive, unconventional viewpoints on nutrition, metabolism, and functional medicine. Special thanks to Dr. Hyman for his early support of my *Manifesto for Thriving in a Mixed-Up World,* and for more than a decade of collaborative friendship.

Ernest Rossi, PhD, for his research and writing on ultradian rhythms; the late Mary Enig, PhD, for her research and writing on fats; and to all the other scientists who have committed themselves to the hard work of figuring out (and helping us understand) how our amazing bodies really work.

Mihaly Csikszentmihalyi, PhD, for his work on flow, for the personal memories he shared of teaching social sciences at Lake Forest College with my dad in the late 1960s, and for helping me place my Healthy Deviant work in a historical and academic context that enriched it substantially.

Arianna Huffington for hiring me to run the Healthy Living vertical at the *Huffington Post* back in 2013 and then generously forgiving me when I realized that job just wasn't for me (in part because this book was already calling out to be written).

Jamie Scott and Anastasia Boulais for grasping the concept of Healthy Deviance straight away, and for inviting me to come speak about it at the Ancestral Health Symposium in New Zealand.

Carl Richards (BehaviorGap.com) for attending that talk in New Zealand

and then referencing my Healthy Deviance work in his *New York Times* column (which turned out to be weirdly important in making it seem "real" to others—and to me, too); and for inspiring the "where to start" Venn diagram in chapter 18.

Mary Jo Kreizer and the University of Minnesota's Earl Bakken Center for Spirituality and Healing for inviting me to speak as part of their Well-Being Lecture Series before this book was published.

Randy Eisenman and Satori Capital for having me come talk about Healthy Deviance as part of their anything-but-conventional corporate wellness initiative and for inspiring my Healthy Deviant Leadership talk.

The Institute for Integrative Nutrition in New York City for giving me a place to share Healthy Deviant ideas with thousands of health coaches and other healthy change agents.

Toni Morrison, Austin Kleon, and a great many wise others for the excellent (and surprisingly difficult-to-follow) advice to "write the book you want to read."

The poet George Mills, my late godfather, for "seeing me" as a kid, taking my adolescent poetry seriously, and helping me regard my creativity as important and inherently worthwhile. George, I thank you for the magical seven-league belt you left in my possession on the night you passed. I am putting it to good use, and I promise to pass it on when I go.

Gary Becker, a family friend (and former student of my dad's) who shared tales from the Lake Forest College days and did a Dad-proxy read of the manuscript that brought tears to my eyes.

My sisters, Andrea and Luisa Gerasimo, and also to Tracy Glenz, Heidi Wachter, Sarah Spencer, Jacque Fletcher, Courtney Helgoe, and Glynnis Lessing (all sisters of a sort) for their early readings and formative discussions of random book-related materials. Special thanks to Maya Bacon for her early read of the manuscript (over margaritas!) and for tolerating me getting up at four in the morning several days running in order to work on this book while we were rooming together at that yoga retreat in Mexico.

To Donna, Gena, Mellie, Jacque, Cindi, Dr. Linda, Dr. Dave, Dr. Josh, Dr. Ren, Cousin Karen, and the whole posse of bodyworkers and healers who helped me keep myself together through good days and rough spots.

The fields, forests, hills, valleys, gardens, ponds, creeks, seeps, and gravel roads of Bubbling Springs Farm, the place of my life and my people, the underlying source and support system for all I do. And to all the land, water, plants, and creatures (seen and unseen) who make my life, and all of our lives, possible.

The generations of Healthy Deviants who came before, with especially deep and wide appreciation to my immigrant ancestors, going all the way back, and to my mother and father, Dorothy Bacon and Jerry Gerasimo, whose open, inquisitive, unconventional, courageous ways of being gave me both reason and freedom to explore many worlds. Thank you, Mom and Dad, for letting me be me, even when I know that must have been tough to watch.

To Jon, my stepfather, and Mike Helfman, my brother-in-law, for joining our family at the perfect time, for keeping things running, and for sticking with us all through thick and thin.

My goofy rescue pit bull pal, Calvin, for the thrice-daily walks, plus runs, zoomies, snuggles, wild ruckuses, and joyous welcomes home. You are the best and most faithful URB buddy ever.

My brilliant, wildly talented friend and partner Alan Bergo (ForagerChef .com) for regularly calling from the kitchen to tell me it's time to stop working and come eat; for making me laugh daily; for lovingly fueling my body-mind with an endless, creative, beautiful array of hand-harvested local, seasonal, foods; and for somehow making me feel worthy of them all.

Finally, deepest thanks and profound respect to all the Healthy Deviants who are embracing the work of making this world a healthier and happier place for all. It will take all of us to dismantle the vicious cycle of the Unhealthy Default Reality. It will take each of us to establish and reinforce the virtuous cycle of Healthy Deviance in all the places we see and feel it lacking. Our work has just begun.

ENDNOTES

Introduction

1 "Wink, Wink, Nudge, Nudge" is a reference to a popular Monty Python sketch of the same title. You kind of have watch the skit to understand: https://youtu.be/4Kwh3R0YjuQ.

Chapter 1

2 C. L. M. Keyes, "The Mental Health Continuum: From Languishing to Flourishing in Life." *Journal of Health and Social Behavior*, 2002; 43: 207–22.

3 Angela Winter, "The Science of Happiness: Barbara Fredrickson on Cultivating Positive Emotions," *The Sun,* May 2009. www.thesunmagazine.org/issues/401/the-science-of -happiness.

4 P. D. Loprinzi, A. Branscum, J. Hanks, and E. Smit, "Healthy Lifestyle Characteristics and Their Joint Association with Cardiovascular Disease Biomarkers in US Adults," *Mayo Clinic Proceeding*s 91, no. 4 (2016): 432–42. doi: 10.1016/j.mayocp.2016.01.009. Epub 2016 Feb 20. www.ncbi.nlm.nih.gov/pubmed/26906650.

5 Linda Searing, "The Big Number: 45 Million Americans Go on a Diet Each Year," *Washington Post,* January 1, 2018, www.washingtonpost.com/national/health-science /the-big-number-45-million-americans-go-on-a-diet-each-year/2017/12/29/04089aec -ebdd-11e7-b698-91d4e35920a3_story.html.

Chapter 2

6 Emily Sohn, "Exercise Is Fundamental to Good Health. So Why Do Few Americans Stick with It?" *Washington Post,* May 7, 2017, www.washingtonpost.com/national/health -science/exercise-is-fundamental-to-good-health-so-why-do-few-americans-stick-with -it/2017/05/05/2c537338-2e81-11e7-8674-437ddb6e813e_story.html. The recommendation for 150 minutes of physical activity comes from the CDC: www.cdc.gov/physicalactivity /basics/adults.

7 The top ten leading causes of death, according to the Centers for Disease Control. www.cdc.gov/nchs/fastats/leading-causes-of-death.htm

8 If you are interested in these topics, I strongly recommend checking out the Ancestral Health Society (www.ancestralhealth.org) and their associated publications, events, and communities.

9   Brandon H. Hidaka, "Depression as a Disease of Modernity: Explanations for Increasing Prevalence," *Journal of Affective Disorders* 140, no. 3 (2012) 205–14, www.ncbi.nlm.nih.gov /pmc/articles/PMC3330161; for more on this, see Stephen Ilardi, PhD, *The Depression Cure.*

10   Many modern-day accidents are tied to fatigue, sleep deprivation, and drug or alcohol intoxication, all of which are tied to modern-day lifestyle patterns and chronic depletion.

11   Awareness of human-caused climate change actually dates back close to a hundred years, but it wasn't until the late 1980s that it started getting regular popular media coverage, and it wasn't until 2006 that the documentary film *An Inconvenient Truth* made it a more widely shared matter of concern. For more on the history of climate change and the science behind it, see the timeline from the American Institute of Physics at https://history.aip .org/climate/timeline.htm.

12   If you want deeper insights on how powerfully advertising drives media, read Gloria Steinem's 1990 essay, "Sex, Lies, and Advertising" available at www1.udel.edu/comm245 /readings/advertising.pdf. Note that the already-blurred line between editorial and advertising has become drastically more blurred since Steinem's essay was originally published three decades ago.

13   www.salon.com/2019/02/01/new-emails-reveal-how-cdc-employees-were-doing-the -bidding-of-coca-cola.

14   If you want more on this topic, consider Michelle Simon's book, *Appetite for Profit: How the Food Industry Undermines Our Health and How to Fight Back*; or Marion Nestle's book, *Food Politics: How the Food Industry Influences Nutrition & Health.*

15   Notwithstanding the current penchant for "community health" and "population health" initiatives (efforts that attempt to more broadly consider and address shared and social determinants of health), the vast majority of our medical dollars are still expended addressing individual health challenges, typically relatively late in their developmental cycle.

Chapter 3

16   R. Moynihan and L. Bero, "Toward a Healthier Patient Voice: More Independence, Less Industry Funding," *JAMA Intern Med.* 177, no. 3 (2017): 350-51. doi:10.1001 /jamainternmed.2016.9179. http://jamanetwork.com/journals/jamainternalmedicine /fullarticle/10.1001/jamainternmed.2016.9179.

17   Although the lack of strong evidence condemning red meats and saturated fats has been at issue for a very long time in nutritional circles, the most recent manifestation comes in a series of research studies reported in the Annals of Internal Medicine and broadcast to the lay public in October 2020 via the New York Times. See "Eat Less Red Meat, Scientists Said. Now Some Believe That Was Bad Advice" (https://www.nytimes. com/2019/09/30/health/red-meat-heart-cancer.html) and "That Perplexing Red Meat Controversy: 5 Things To Know" (https://www.nytimes.com/2019/09/30/health /red-meat-questions-answers.html).

18   As of this book's printing, the Mayo Clinic website (www.mayoclinic.org/healthy-lifestyle /nutrition-and-healthy-eating/expert-answers/butter-vs-margarine/faq-20058152) was still suggesting margarine "usually tops butter" when it comes to heart health (see text below). It was also suggesting that you "limit the amount you use to limit the calories." Harvard's site (www.health.harvard.edu/staying-healthy/butter-vs-margarine) also sug- gests that "healthier alternatives" to butter include "vegetable oil–based spreads." It goes on to suggest: "Next time you tear into a warm loaf of bread or roll, consider dipping it in olive oil rather than coating it in butter. If you're trying to lower your cholesterol, stanol-based spreads (for example, Benecol and Take Control) are even better, since

regular use can help lower LDL cholesterol levels." Both the promotion of grain-based breads and the suggestion that brand-name processed products are "better than" natural, traditional, whole-food-based options like butter and olive oil are common themes in conventional health media. From the Mayo Clinic's website: "Which spread is better for my heart—butter or margarine?" Katherine Zeratsky, RD, LD, says, "Margarine usually tops butter when it comes to heart health. Margarine is made from vegetable oils, so it contains unsaturated 'good' fats—polyunsaturated and monounsaturated fats. These types of fats help reduce low-density lipoprotein (LDL), or 'bad,' cholesterol when substituted for saturated fat. Butter, on the other hand, is made from animal fat, so it contains more saturated fat. But not all margarines are created equal—some margarines contain trans fat. In general, the more solid the margarine, the more trans fat it contains. So stick margarines usually have more trans fat than tub margarines do. Trans fat, like saturated fat, increases blood cholesterol levels and the risk of heart disease. In addition, trans fat lowers high-density lipoprotein (HDL), or 'good,' cholesterol levels. So skip the stick and opt for soft or liquid margarine instead. Look for a spread that doesn't have trans fats and has the least amount of saturated fat. When comparing spreads, be sure to read the Nutrition Facts panel and check the grams of saturated fat and trans fat."

19 As of this book's printing, the version of the National Diabetes Prevention Protocol Participant Notebook that I've referenced here was available for download at https://www.cdc.gov/diabetes/prevention/pdf/handouts.pdf. I can only hope that it will soon be radically revised and updated. The American Diabetes Association convened in late 2018 to update their consensus statement on nutrition, and for the first time signaled an important shift in their willingness to embrace lower-carbohydrate and higher-fat eating approaches for pre-diabetic and diabetic individuals. In April 2019, they published a report ("Nutrition Therapy for Adults with Prediabetes or Diabetes: A Consensus Report") that quietly reflected these important changes (it is currently available for download at http://care.diabetesjournals.org/content/diacare/early/2019/04/10 /dci19-0014.full.pdf). However, no alarms were sounded, no major consensus-reversal announcements were made, and no public re-education campaign was launched. So, given the pro-grain, anti-fat brainwashing that our entire country has experienced over the past 30 years, I fear it will take decades before many mainstream health-education resources will be updated accordingly, and before most conventional health practitioners begin offering advice in keeping with current science. And if history is any indication, it will be longer still before any of the supposedly authoritative sources who have been aggressively pushing ill-founded, damaging dietary counsel at taxpayer expense will openly admit "we were wrong."

20 Note that the word *ego*, in this context, doesn't refer to having "a big ego" or thinking highly of yourself; it just refers to the part of your psyche that—in Freud's lingo of the *id*, *ego*, and *superego*—controls your rational thinking and decision making.

21 There has been some debate in recent years about just how reliable this conclusion is. As noted in this article from *Slate*, recent studies using tightly controlled computer-testing models do not reliably produce the same results that have been borne out through decades of previous peer-reviewed research using more complex and realistic conditions. However, computer-testing models are not real life. If you have doubts concerning the science on ego depletion, I encourage you to read deeper into the details of how these more recent studies were conducted. Based on the evidence I've reviewed, I remain convinced that the original studies on ego depletion are more reflective of real-life circumstances, and thus more useful. Similarly, the studies on Self-Directed Therapy yield important conclusions (applicable to real-life) about why certain scenarios and decisions prove ego-depleting for some and intrinsically motivating for others. This research is consistent with my own experience as a Healthy Deviant, in which most healthy choices (like "just saying no" to candy or soda, for example) are not at all difficult or draining, and in which choosing

to take a walk rather than watch television requires no "discipline" at all. See www.slate
.com/articles/health_and_science/cover_story/2016/03/ego_depletion_an_influential
_theory_in_psychology_may_have_just_been_debunked.html.

22   May Lwin, Maureen Morrin, Stanley W. H. Tang, Jin Yong Low, Thu Nguyen, and Wei Xun
     Lee, "See the Seal? Understanding Restrained Eaters' Responses to Nutritional Messages on
     Food Packaging," *Health Communication* 29 (2013), 10.1080/10410236.2013.789131, www.
     researchgate.net/publication/258101387_See_the_Seal_Understanding_Restrained_Eat-
     ers'_Responses_to_Nutritional_Messages_on_Food_Packaging.

23   A famed NASA researcher, James Wise, PhD, once explained to me that the most stress-
     reducing human-designed environments tend to very closely mimic, in mathematical
     terms, the fractal complexity of the African savannah, where our genetically determined
     preferences were first formed. Our modern environments tend to be either massively more
     cluttered (think Dollar Store) or more plain (think institutional and modern-minimalist
     interiors) and decidedly *non*-fractal, contributing to system-wide stress on the human
     body-mind. For more on this, see Wise's paper "The Quantitative Modelling of Human
     Spatial Habitability" (https://ntrs.nasa.gov/archive/nasa/casi.ntrs.nasa.gov/19890006159
     .pdf). See also the paper by Nikos A. Salingaros, "Fractal Art and Architecture Reduce
     Physiological Stress," which references Wise's and other researchers' work.

24   There's a fast-growing collection of research showing that various aspects of mood, atti-
     tude, and central nervous system function are directly impacted by the balance of flora
     in our intestinal tract. For more on this, see the studies of how mice with healthier gut
     flora responded to forced-swim "despair" scenarios (https://www.nature.com/articles
     /srep43859). Worth noting is that the connection works both ways: Being stressed and
     depressed negatively influences your microbiome, and a disrupted microbiome also
     negatively affects mood and mental function.

25   Studies show that if you have a depleted immune system because you are fighting off a
     cold or cancer, your willpower can be affected.

Chapter 4

26   Ivana Buric, Miguel Farias, Jonathan Jong, Christopher Mee, and Inti A. Brazil, "What
     Is the Molecular Signature of Mind–Body Interventions? A Systematic Review of
     Gene Expression Changes Induced by Meditation and Related Practices," *Frontiers in
     Immunology*, 2017; 8 DOI: 10.3389/fimmu.2017.00670.

27   As described in Mihaly Csikszentmihalyi, *Flow: The Psychology of Optimal Experience*
     (New York: HarperCollins, 1990).

28   You find yourself standing in the potato chip aisle? Okay, how did you get there? Where
     on your Trouble Clock are you right now, and what preceded this moment or set it
     up? What's going to happen next? Put your attention on every detail of the scene. The
     lights, the smells, the colorful packages, the sound of bags crinkling, of music playing, of
     shopping carts going by. Snap into high-definition awareness and curiosity about what
     is happening in your body-mind, in that aisle in that market, in that moment. Be keenly
     interested in the potential of the moment. What if you reach out for a package but don't
     grab it. What if you grab it, and put it back? What if you eat the chips? What if you don't?
     What if you eat one and throw the rest of the bag away? What if you plan to eat just a few
     and then find you can't stop? Can you stay awake for this entire experience, whatever it
     is? Can you observe it without judgment, or notice the judgment that is coming up? Can
     you notice the exact moment when you are losing it and about to go unconscious? Can
     you be present even in the reaction that comes afterward? Keep your attention engaged
     at that level of self-monitoring fascination for long enough, and you will find you are in
     a form of "flow."

29   As a rule, the longer your body has been "pissed off," and the more resultant damage done to your biology, the longer it will take to heal that damage, but it's often only a matter of days before the first noticeable signs of healing appear. Many integrative and naturopathic health professionals have observed that the body tends to heal "from the inside out and from the top down." If you accept that notion, it stands to reason that healthy skin and healthy feet tend to be good indicators that the body as a whole is reasonably happy. That said, it is entirely possible to have healthy-looking skin, healthy-looking feet, and still have a tumor growing or a blood-clot lurking somewhere within you, so it's best not to get overconfident about how well you are doing just on the basis of those two factors.

Chapter 13

30   For more on the contrast between "fixed" and "growth" mindsets, see Carol Dweck, *Mindset,* and her TED Talk on the subject, or visit her site at www.mindsetonline.com.

Chapter 15

31   Learn about Eric Garland, PhD, LCSW, and his mind-body therapeutic method (Mindfulness-Oriented Recovery Enhancement, or M.O.R.E) at https://drericgarland.com.

32   A. Babar, N. A. Al-Wabel, S. Shams, A. Ahamad, S. A. Khan, and F. Anwar, "Essential Oils Used in Aromatherapy: A Systemic Review," *Asian Pacific Journal of Tropical Biomedicine* 5, no. 8 (2015): 601–11, www.sciencedirect.com/science/article/pii/S2221169115001033.

Chapter 16

33   See appendix for resources related to breaks, ultradian rhythms, productivity, and ego depletion.

Chapter 18

34   Hat tip to Dan and Chip Heath for their terrific book *Switch: How to Change When Change is Hard* and also to Jon Tierney and Roy Baumeister for insights from their very helpful book, *Willpower,* which while I did not always agree with, I do very much respect. I have read, realistically, a thousand other books on behavior change, healthy habits, Positive Psychology, and related topics, and my thoughts and opinions have been formed by all of them. I stand on the shoulders of giants in this regard, and owe a huge debt of gratitude to the researchers, teachers, writers, experimenters, monks, mystics, medicine-people, and other rabble-rousers who have taught me all I know.

35   Some of the most exciting research in this area shows we can develop the neurocircuitry that supports self-regulated decision making and behavior by practicing on less daunting willpower challenges. For example, smoking-cessation research showing smokers who were given exercises to help them build self-regulatory steam in advance of quitting smoking were three times as likely to succeed in kicking the habit.

36   Although I think most of us could stand to eat a greater quantity and variety of vegetables than we do, I am not a fan of the push toward vegan and vegetarian diets on the basis of health, or on the basis of environmental responsibility. My reasons for this could fill a book. They have, in fact, filled several excellent and meticulously researched books by other writers, including Lierre Keith, former vegan and author of *The Vegetarian Myth,* and journalist Nina Teicholz, author of *Big Fat Surprise.* That said, I understand and respect that many eaters choose low-meat or meat-free diets out of ethical opposition to factory-farmed meat production and animal cruelty—an opposition that I whole-heartedly share. Industrial-scale farming of both plants and animals is inherently toxic, wasteful, and destructive. With this in mind, I encourage all ethically concerned and health-motivated eaters to support small, local, responsible farmers, especially those who are raising animals on pasture and rebuilding soil in ways that support healthy

bodies, healthy ecosystems, sustainable local economies, and a stable planet. The path of Healthy Deviance (which involves experimenting to see what works and doesn't work for you) is a path that can and must be open to all, including those who consume animal products and those who choose to avoid them. I would, however, contend that most people will enjoy far better health and vitality—particularly over the long haul—as the result of including reasonable quantities of carefully sourced animal products in their diets. I also believe that our planet's ecological future will be better served through the support of small-scale, sustainable animal husbandry (all of which is inherently "plant based") than by industrial, fossil-fuel-based mono-cropping of vegetables and grains. Full disclosure: I was raised and still live on a small family farm where we raise a lot of our own food, including rotationally grazed, pastured animals. If you want to hear more about my views on this topic, please listen to the "Eating Meat" episode of *The Living Experiment* podcast, available at www.livingexperiment.com.

37   Stuart Wolpert, "Dieting Does Not Work, UCLA Researchers Report," *UCLA Newsroom,* April 3, 2007, http://newsroom.ucla.edu/releases/Dieting-Does-Not-Work-UCLA -Researchers-7832.

38   Anahad O'Connor, "The Key to Weight Loss Is Diet Quality, Not Quantity, a New Study Finds," *New York Times,* February 20, 2018, www.nytimes.com/2018/02/20/well/eat /counting-calories-weight-loss-diet-dieting-low-carb-low-fat.html.

39   E. M. Steele, L. G. Baraldi, M. Louzada, J.-C. Moubarac, D. Mozaffarian, and C. A. Monteiro, "Ultra-Processed Foods and Added Sugars in the U.S. Diet: Evidence from a Nationally Representative Cross-Sectional Study," *BMJ Open,* 2016, https://bmjopen.bmj.com /content/6/3/e009892.

40   Henry Bodkin, "Alzheimer's Could Be Caused by Excess Sugar: New Study Finds 'Molecular Link,' " *Telegraph,* February 23, 2017, www.telegraph.co.uk/science/2017/02/23 /alzheimers-could-caused-excess-sugar-new-study-finds-molecular.

41   Olga Khazan, "The Startling Link Between Sugar and Alzheimer's," *The Atlantic,* January 26, 2018, www.theatlantic.com/health/archive/2018/01/the-startling-link-between-sugar -and-alzheimers/551528.

Chapter 19

42   A. S. Heller, A. S. Fox, et al., "The Neurodynamics of Affect in the Laboratory Predicts Persistence of Real-World Emotional Responses, *Journal of Neuroscience* 35, no. 29 (2015): 10503–09, www.jneurosci.org/content/35/29/10503.

43   Eric Garland's articles on savoring: https://drericgarland.com/tag/savoring.

Chapter 20

44   I borrowed this phrase directly from the teachings of Lafayette Morehouse, where I've taken a number of fascinating courses over the years. I owe them a debt of gratitude for many other helpful perspectives and points of view. You can hear my interviews with Morehouse faculty members in four separate episodes of *The Living Experiment* podcast ("Winning Cycles," "Intimacy and Connection," "Win-Win Relating," and "Resistance to Pleasure") available at www.livingexperiment.com.

Chapter 21

45   A phrase borrowed from Master Kan, a fictional Zen martial-arts master who patiently schools his young Shaolin monk disciple, Caine (a.k.a. "Grasshopper"), in the classic 1970s television program, *Kung Fu.*

46   Functional, integrative, and naturopathic medicine approaches tend to be much better at resolving chronic conditions, but they are often not covered by conventional health

insurance. They also require you to make changes to your daily habits, including food, movement, sleep, and stress management.

Chapter 22

47 For the complete text of Dr. King's speech, see: https://thesocietypages.org/toolbox /dr-martin-luther-king-jr-social-scientists.

INDEX

Numbered Terms

ABOUT THE AUTHOR

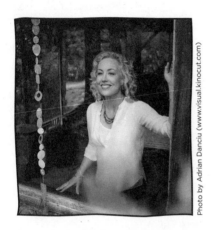

Photo by Adrian Danciu (www.visual.kinocut.com)

PILAR GERASIMO is an award-winning health journalist and founding editor of *Experience Life* magazine, a healthy-living print publication that reaches more than three million people worldwide. She is also co-host (with Whole30 cofounder Dallas Hartwig) of the top-rated podcast *The Living Experiment.* Pilar has served as top health editor for *The Huffington Post*, chief creative officer for the Institute for Integrative Nutrition, and as a strategic advisor for Brian Johnson's Optimize Enterprises. She lectures at universities and leads workshops at retreat centers like Kripalu, Omega Institute, Sundance, 1440 Multiversity, and Rancho La Puerta. She has appeared as an expert guest with Dr. Oz on Oprah & Friends Radio, CBS, NBC, and CBS television affiliates, and on Mayo Clinic TV. She also consults with organizations to help them encourage and empower the Healthy Deviants within their ranks. Pilar lives on an organic family farm in Wisconsin with Calvin, her irrepressible rescue pit bull pal. Learn more at PilarGerasimo.com and HealthyDeviant.com.

ABOUT NORTH ATLANTIC BOOKS

North Atlantic Books (NAB) is an independent, nonprofit publisher committed to a bold exploration of the relationships between mind, body, spirit, and nature. Founded in 1974, NAB aims to nurture a holistic view of the arts, sciences, humanities, and healing. To make a donation or to learn more about our books, authors, events, and newsletter, please visit www.northatlanticbooks.com.

North Atlantic Books is the publishing arm of the Society for the Study of Native Arts and Sciences, a 501(c)(3) nonprofit educational organization that promotes cross-cultural perspectives linking scientific, social, and artistic fields. To learn how you can support us, please visit our website.